2004

Organization Ethics in Health Care

Organization Ethics in Health Care

EDWARD M. SPENCER
ANN E. MILLS
MARY V. RORTY
PATRICIA H. WERHANE

New York   Oxford
OXFORD UNIVERSITY PRESS
2000

Oxford University Press

Oxford   New York
Athens   Auckland   Bangkok   Bogotá   Buenos Aires   Calcutta
Cape Town   Chennai   Dar es Salaam   Delhi   Florence   Hong Kong   Istanbul
Karachi   Kuala Lumpur   Madrid   Melbourne   Mexico City   Mumbai
Nairobi   Paris   São Paulo   Singapore   Taipei   Tokyo   Toronto   Warsaw

and associated companies in
Berlin   Ibadan

Copyright © 2000 by Oxford University Press, Inc.

Published by Oxford University Press, Inc.,
198 Madison Avenue, New York, New York, 10016

Oxford is a registered trademark of Oxford University Press

Library of Congress Cataloging-in-Publication Data
Spencer, Edward M.
Organization ethics in health care /
Edward M. Spencer . . . [et al.].
p.   cm.   Includes bibliographical references and index.
ISBN 0-19-512980-6
1. Managed care plans (Medical care)—Moral and ethical aspects.
2. Medical ethics.
3. Corporate culture—Moral and ethical aspects.
I. Title.
[DNLM: 1. Ethics, Medical.
2. Health Facilities—organization & administration.
3. Organizational Culture.
W 50 S745o 2000]   RA413.S64 2000   174'.2—dc21
DNLM/DLC   for Library of Congress   99-31080

9 8 7 6 5 4 3 2

Printed in the United States of America
on acid-free paper

Preface

This book represents a new approach to healthcare ethics. Unlike previous alternative approaches to ethics in health care, we are advocating a focus on the ethics of the entire organization, a focus that encompasses and integrates the resources and activities of clinical ethics, business ethics, the ethics of healthcare management, and professional ethics within the organization. This inclusive perspective we call "organization ethics."

Although we will discuss managed care organizations (MCOs) and health maintenance organizations (HMOs), the primary subject of this book will be medium-sized and large organizations that provide health services. We start with provider organizations, because many of these healthcare organizations (HCOs) have well-established institutional clinical ethics committees that deal with ethical issues in patient care. Thus thinking about ethical issues on an institutional level is not alien to HCOs even if these ethics committees have not concentrated specifically on business, professional, or organizational issues. If provider organizations can create organization ethics programs that integrate clinical, medical, professional, and economic perspectives while delivering high-quality health services, such organizations will serve as models for MCOs, HMOs, preferred provider organizations (PPOs), and other organizations in the business of purveying, funding, and, in some instances, delivering healthcare services.

The book is both a theoretical analysis of the ethics of healthcare organizations and a guide to how, in practice, a viable, robust, inclusive ethics program can be developed within a healthcare organization. Thus the audience for the book is not merely those who teach healthcare ethics and healthcare administration, and their students. The book is also written for practicing healthcare administrators and professionals who struggle daily with ethical issues in managing and providing health care to a patient population in community settings where demands for high-quality health care is acute. Teachers using the book in the classroom will find the philosophical dimensions of organization ethics important for students. Practicing healthcare managers and professionals may well want to focus their attention on chapters 9–12 of the book, where the practical implications of our thesis are worked out in some detail.

Chapters 1 through 5 of the book introduce our thesis and discuss questions of organizational ethics, and the limitations of clinical ethics, business ethics, and professional ethics to address many of the recent changes in the HCO and the relationships among its key stakeholders. Chapters 6 and 7 describe the historical development of the HCO and explore the external environment in which the HCO is operating today. Chapters 8 through 11, discusses the internal ethical climate of the HCO. This part of the book offers detailed recommendations for the implementation of a successful organization ethics program. A more detailed description of each chapter follows.

Chapter 1 introduces the reader to the concept of organization ethics and looks at some of the initiatives that important regulatory and representative groups have made in that direction. We begin to differentiate our approach to organization ethics in this chapter.

Because this is a book about organization *ethics,* in Chapter 2 we outline further what we mean by ethics, and introduce the reader to some prominent ethical theories. We then shift attention from individuals to organizations. We deal with the question of organizational roles and role morality, and suggest how one can hold an organization, as well as the individuals who constitute it, morally responsible.

Chapter 3 focuses on patient care or clinical ethics. We trace its roots in bioethics and medical ethics and explain how its use of casuistry is an effective approach in dealing with ethics issues in HCOs. While institutional ethics committees are by and large clinically focused, we argue that that framework can be reconceptualized in thinking about organization ethics committees. Chapter 4 addresses business ethics. There we discuss the limitations of a model that suggests that a manager's responsibility is primarily to shareholders, and we reformulate that responsibility in terms of the mission of a HCO. We then reframe normative stakeholder theory to take into account the unique priorities of HCOs, and their complex accountability relationships.

Chapter 5 concentrates on professional ethics. We show that while the professions, like HCOs, prioritize patient care as their primary concern, most professional associations have yet to think through implications of healthcare organizations for their professionals, most of whom are now employees as well. The challenge is to capture the professional priority of the value-creating activity of providing patient care in an organizational setting.

Chapters 6 and 7 discuss the historical development of healthcare organizations in the United States, the external social, religious, technological, and political climates in which they grew and were changed, and the present-day state of affairs in health care in the United States. We identify in these chapters four distinct shifts in the HCO's orientation. We argue that all but the last shift has occurred within the context of values that have been articulated and endorsed by society. These chapters are important to students of health care to give them a context within which to comprehend the healthcare situation in the United States as we move into the new millenium. Many readers will be familiar with the history of the HCO and may be tempted to gloss over these chapters. However, we believe our conceptualization of it supports our earlier theoretical contentions.

Given the theoretical background developed in the early chapters and the historical, political, social and technological context out of which health care is delivered today (Chapters 6 and 7), the reader is then prepared to begin thinking about how ethics, ethics programs, and ethics committees can make a difference in healthcare organizations, and why such initiatives are crucial for the future survival and flourishing of health care. Chapter 8 begins this task by analyzing how an HCO can develop a positive internal ethical climate given today's social, political, and market forces. Chapter 9 outlines the nuts-and-bolts task of instituting an organization ethics program within an HCO. Given those recommendations, in Chapter 10 we focus on issues in quality, compliance, and risk management as ancillary problems for an organization ethics program. Finally, in Chapter 11, we discuss questions concerning evaluation of the program and its activities.

Developing an organization ethics program that is truly mission driven, that integrates all aspects of the HCO, and that creates a positive ethical climate that drives values-based decision making is truly a daunting endeavor. But, we will conclude, it is worth the effort. Trust of HCOs and in the managers and the professionals who work there will be reinvigorated and the issues of financing and delivery of health care can be dealt with adequately within the context of a well-articulated and broadly agreed upon mission and positive ethical climate. Organization ethics is an important challenge to HCOs and all who work in the healthcare arena. How this industry and the healthcare professions respond to this challenge will determine the course of health care in the United States for the foreseeable future.

This project has been supported by the Olsson Center for Applied Ethics in the Darden Graduate School of Business Administration and the Center for Biomedical Ethics in the School of Medicine, both at the University of Virginia. In particular we thank Jonathan D. Moreno and R. Edward Freeman for their encouragement. We also are gratefully appreciative of the Ethics Institute at the American Medical Association for providing a think tank to generate some of these ideas. We wish to express our deep appreciation and gratitude to Carlton Haywood Jr., our student and intern, who has assisted us in the preparation of this manuscript. Our appreciation and thanks as well to Emily G. Powell and Karen F. Musselman. In addition, the book has benefited from discussions we have had with hundreds of students, academics in applied ethics, and practicing healthcare professionals and managers who are concerned about the present and the future state of healthcare delivery in this country. The editors at Oxford University Press, in particular Jeffrey House and Charles Annis, have encouraged and supported the genesis and delivery of this book. Its shortcomings are our own.

Charlottesville, Virginia   E. M. S.
April 1999   A. E. M.
                                                              M. V. R.
                                                              P. H. W

Contents

Organization Ethics in Health Care

1

The Background for Organization Ethics

Scrutiny of the ethical operations of larger non-healthcare-related corporations is not new. Beginning shortly after the Watergate scandal, both governmental watchdog agencies and private groups have been showing an increasing interest in how corporations address ethical issues. Recent specific cases of ethically problematic activities in a number of corporations have received particular attention and criticism, and, within the corporations themselves, have led to the development of compliance and ethics programs as attempts to meet the criticism. Originally, the mission of these programs was not always focused on the ethical climate of the organization or on the details of the decision making process within the organization. Rather, illegal activities such as fraud, improper handling of funds, unscrupulous practices, or overtly immoral behavior (usually sexual harassment issues) constituted the majority of cases of concern. Such programs that developed along these lines were more clearly compliance programs than ethics programs, although they were often labeled "ethics." The aim of a compliance program is to make sure a company complies with regulations, laws, and those societal norms for which there is general consensus. The aim of an ethics program is to develop and evaluate the organizational mission, to create a positive ethical climate within the organization that perpetuates the mission, to develop decision models for insuring this perpetuation as reflected in organizational activities, and to serve as a cheerleader, evaluator, and critic of organizational, professional, and managerial

3

behavior. Compliance is part of that, since disobeying the law or circumventing regulations is ordinarily not considered appropriate moral or legal behavior. However, an ethics program is broader and its mandates less clear-cut than compliance.

Recently, corporate compliance and ethics programs have been encouraged by the federal government with its advancement of the Federal Sentencing Guidelines for corporations. These guidelines specify appropriate sentences for individuals and institutions found guilty of specific criminal activity. Because sentences under these guidelines can be mitigated when the guilty organization can demonstrate that it has in place a "effective program within the organization which seeks to deter and prevent criminal activity" (Federal Sentencing Guidelines, 1995a), most corporations have begun such activities under the rubrics of "corporate compliance programs" and "ethics programs."

Until the recent increase in attention to HCOs by federal authorities, ethics programs in those institutions had been primarily focused on ethical issues related to the care of individual patients. Since the late 1980s and early 1990s, the missions of most HCOs' institutional ethics committees have been to protect the rights of the individual patient. Before this, healthcare regulators and accrediting agencies saw the institutional ethics committee, along with Medicare and Medicaid regulations affecting patient care, as adequate protection for the patient, leaving HCOs with little to fear from the Justice Department. Consideration of ethical issues outside the patient care and research arenas was mainly restricted to employee relations, for which there were often specific contracts, policies, and guidelines required by law.

As HCOs, MCOs, HMOs, and other healthcare payers and providers have grown and become increasingly complex, they have begun to receive more negative attention from the Justice Department, with particular emphasis on nonadherence to Medicare and Medicaid regulations, leading to questions of potential fraud or other criminally liable activities. The advent and rapid market penetration of managed care has increased this scrutiny. The Justice Department is now looking at HCOs' compliance to government regulations as well as their obedience to laws, thereby assuring the application of sentencing guidelines in the healthcare industry just as they have been applied in other industries. It has now become clear that HCOs need a mechanism to respond to externally imposed regulations and requirements affecting institutional operations, requirements that have only recently begun to be relevant in the healthcare arena. HCOs have also become more aware of the ethical issues related to their business functions. This response mechanism is being called "organization ethics" and is already an important primary responsibility of the HCO; a responsibility that, if ignored, can harm the HCO, both as a business and as a healthcare provider.

With Justice Department attention as a stimulus, larger HCOs and healthcare systems, like non-healthcare-related corporations, have instituted or are considering instituting a corporate compliance program or an organization ethics program in hopes of mitigating any potential sentences under sentencing guidelines. Specific fines required by sentencing guidelines may be decreased up to 95 percent (HFMA Express News, 1997) because of the presence and demonstrated activity of a compliance or ethics program that meets federal standards. This constitutes a strong reason for HCOs to develop and maintain such activities.

WHAT IS ORGANIZATION ETHICS?

In its simplest terms, organization ethics is the articulation, application, and evaluation of the consistent values and moral positions of an organization by which it is defined, both internally and externally. This process of articulation, application, and evaluation has been developed and maintained in other businesses under the rubric of "total ethics management," a concept rooted in the understanding of organizations as systems (Navran, 1997). Within the healthcare arena, accrediting organizations such as the Joint Commission for Accreditation of Healthcare Organizations (JCAHO)* have broadly defined organization ethics as those aspects of the operation of the HCO that have to do with the "ethical responsibility" of the organization itself "to conduct its business and patient care practices in an honest, decent and proper manner" (Joint Commission for Accreditation of Healthcare Organizations, 1997, p. RI 24). A process-oriented definition of organization ethics, and one to which we subscribe, was advanced by the Virginia Bioethics Network (VBN).† It states: "Organization ethics consists of a process(es) to address ethical issues associated with the business, financial, and management areas of healthcare organizations, as well as with professional, educational, and contractual relationships affecting the operation of the HCO" (See Appendix 1 for complete text of VBN organization ethics guidelines). These processes include articulation, application, and evaluation of the organization's mission statement. This definition demands that organization ethics activities encompass all aspects of the operation of the HCO so that a positive ethical climate can be developed and maintained.

Organizational "ethical climate" consists of the shared perceptions of the "general and pervasive characteristics of [an] organization [of a system] affecting a

---

*The Joint Commission for Accreditation of Healthcare Organizations (JCAHO) is a private, nonprofit, quasi-official accrediting organization representing five professional groups: American Medical Association, American Hospital Association, American College of Physicians, American College of Surgeons, and American Dental Association.

†The Virginia Bioethics Network is a self-supporting, self-directed group of healthcare organizations (including hospitals, nursing homes, home health agencies, managed-care organizations, and regional bioethics networks) with patient care ethics committees, which have joined together to advance ethics activities in health care. VBN has developed "Guidelines" addressing both patient care ethics programs in healthcare organizations and organization ethics issues.

broad range of decisions" (Victor & Cullen, 1988, p. 101). Ethical climate defines the organization in both its internal and external relationships and permeates the whole. It is articulated via value statements, mission statements, organization codes of ethics, policies addressing specific ethical issues, and most importantly, through its effect on the attitudes and activities of everyone associated with the organization. Obviously, then, one could create or perpetuate a negative or a positive ethical climate in any organization. A positive ethical climate has at least two important characteristics. First, it is an organizational culture where the mission and vision of the organization are consistent with its expectations for professional and managerial performance and consistent with the goals of the organization as they are actually practiced. Second, a positive ethical climate is one that embodies a set of values that reflect societal norms for what organizations should value, how they should prioritize their mission, vision, and goals, and how they and their professionals and managers should behave. The aim of an organization ethics program is to produce a positive ethical climate where the organizational policies, activities, and self-evaluation mechanisms integrate patient, business, and professional perspectives in consistent and positive value-creating activities that articulate, apply, and reinforce its mission. Demonstrating how to achieve such an organizational climate is the purpose of this book.

ORGANIZATION ETHICS IN HEALTHCARE ORGANIZATIONS

Although the fear of Justice Department investigations provides some stimulus, to date the major force for calling attention to organization ethics by HCOs has been the JCAHO and its promulgation of standards directly addressing organization ethics. In 1995, with no fanfare and without much prior discussion with the HCOs it accredits, the JCAHO added a section called "Organization Ethics" to its accreditation standards for all types of HCOs. These standards focused the attention of the HCOs on a particular set of issues which had not been fully addressed by the usual healthcare regulatory mechanisms. Subsequent expansion of the scope of these new standards has made it clear that the JCAHO is serious about organization ethics. Accredited HCOs are expected to address these issues in several specific ways:

1. By developing and instituting an organization code of ethics which addresses a number of specific activities of the HCO including billing, patient transfer, marketing, etc;
2. By addressing, specifically, ethical issues in contractual obligations; and
3. By addressing ethical issues in professional relationships, both within and beyond the HCO for Accreditation of Healthcare Organizations, (Joint Commission, 1997, pp. RI-24–RI-32).

The JCAHO states that its mission is to improve the quality of health care provided to the public, and it attempts to fulfill this mission by providing healthcare accreditation and related services that support performance improvement in HCOs. The JCAHO evaluates and accredits more than 15,000 HCOs in the United States. JCAHO accreditation, or equivalent accreditation from another accrediting agency, is a requirement for Medicaid and Medicare reimbursement, thus representing a strong financial incentive for HCOs to maintain JCAHO accreditation and thereby necessitating attention to organization ethics requirements for JCAHO accreditation. Recently, JCAHO inspectors involved in the periodic inspections required for continued accreditation have been focusing on the organization ethics standards. They have lowered accreditation scores for individual HCOs if they have not found evidence that the HCO has given full attention to these standards.

In response to Justice Department attention to HCOs and to the JCAHO organization ethics standards, the American Hospital Association (AHA) has developed an "Organizational Ethics Initiative" (American Hospital Association, 1997). In 1997, the AHA, the largest and most influential hospital organization in the United States, began a pilot educational program aimed at fostering the development of organizational ethics in all of its member institutions. Introducing this initiative, the AHA states:

> As leaders of healthcare organizations, we believe that it is crucial that we establish ethical guideposts that will help us guide our business and governance practices, while maintaining our accountability to the communities we serve. Common sense is not enough. It is clear today that the ethical thing to do cannot be taken for granted and that many stakeholders in the healthcare system do not share, or give meaning to, certain core values. Accordingly, AHA has chosen to serve as the catalyst by encouraging its members and others providing healthcare, to adopt initiatives which will foster both compliance and ethics in their individual institutions. We believe such programs would invigorate and strengthen the covenant of trust between healthcare organizations and the communities they serve. (American Hospital Association, 1997)

This initiative represents a commitment on the part of the AHA to support its members in making organization ethics an integral part of the HCO at all levels. The AHA's Organization Ethics Initiative consists of educational workshops and consultation from experts with experience in developing ethics programs in other industries. Consultation is available throughout the various stages of development of each participating HCO's organization ethics activities. The AHA states,

> To be truly successful, an organization ethics initiative must be internalized at all levels throughout an institution or system and provide open avenues for communication, dialogue, feedback, and training. Such an effort takes time and the commitment of the CEO and other hospital leaders to model critical values and behaviors in their own actions formally and informally. Ultimately, the effectiveness of any or-

ganizational ethics initiative is inexorably tied to the concrete, observable behaviors and decisions of a healthcare institution's management and professional staff. (American Hospital Association, 1997, p. 3)

GOALS OF THE ORGANIZATION ETHICS INITIATIVE ARTICULATED BY THE AHA ARE:

1. Help provide healthcare executives with some of the tools and information helpful in achieving the Ethical Policies ratified by the Board of Governors of the American College of Healthcare Executives
2. Develop and communicate the vital importance of organizational ethics for healthcare providers throughout the U.S.
3. Identify and cultivate healthcare leaders who are personally and professionally committed to fostering organizational ethics within healthcare institutions and systems
4. Engage healthcare leadership in the process of determining their organizational ethics needs in terms of tools, training, and resources
5. Create tools, training, and resources to integrate values into the normal channels of management, decision making, and every other organizational activity
6. Gather models of what other organizations or industries have done to create systems and structures which are designed to support and reinforce their values
7. Provide training for CEOs, Trustees, and other healthcare leaders throughout the institution or system to ensure that they have the guidelines, skills, knowledge, and competency to make ethically sound decisions on a day-to-day basis
8. Work with the leadership of healthcare organizations in the promotion and exchange of information and experience among colleagues to resolve ethical questions and dilemmas (American Hospital Association, 1997, p. 4)

There is little doubt that organization ethics in some form will be a part of HCOs and healthcare systems of the future. Exactly what this will mean and how it will be addressed in each HCO or system is still an open question. The positions of the JCAHO and the AHA, although compatible, focus on different aspects of healthcare ethics. The JCAHO is more concerned with the effects of the organization's activities on individual patient care. The AHA focuses on the HCO as a business entity and applies business ethics principles to the HCO. We believe both these perspectives are important. However, we do not believe either initiative is likely to be able to fulfill the stated goals unless the perspective on organization ethics is widened. This book represents an effort to do so.

DISTINGUISHING CHARACTERISTICS
OF HEALTHCARE ORGANIZATIONS

A *healthcare organization*, as we will use the term in this book, is a medium-sized or large provider organization with an administrative structure consisting of a board of directors, management personnel, and professionals, and which supplies one or more healthcare interventions and services to individual patients and groups of patients. Common examples are hospitals, nursing homes, home health agencies, and healthcare systems. Managed care organizations that have a patient care function can be considered HCOs; otherwise we will consider them as administrative organizations. HCOs are made up of healthcare professionals, managers, and other employees. They are responsible for patient and population health care, they have obligations to the healthcare insurers who ordinarily are not patients themselves, and they have duties to the communities in which they operate and serve. To be effective, organization ethics for HCOs must encompass a number of ethical perspectives, allowing and encouraging business, professional, and clinical imperatives to maintain their traditional stances when they can contribute positively to the ethical climate of the HCO. How that is to be accomplished requires that we are clear about the distinguishing features of HCOs.

HCOs are unlike other, non-healthcare-related businesses and organizations in several ways: they are not identical to healthcare professional associations; as organizations they are distinct from the professionals who provide medical care in these and other settings; and they are unlike other social organizations that provide specific beneficial services for their clients.

As businesses, HCOs are distinctive in that the payer for services, be it an employer, governmental agency, or insurance company, is commonly not the "consumer" of the service provided. This means the major decisions about access to, and cost of, healthcare interventions are at least partially made by an entity that may be more interested in cost distributions than in the availability and quality of interventions for individual patients. In some instances the patient, as recipient, has little clout to affect the availability of particular healthcare professionals from whom she can seek care. Nor can she be assured that she will have access to particular treatments and interventions, even though these interventions and treatments may be of proven value. In addition, patients are often vulnerable because of their illness. This vulnerability and the lack of the requisite knowledge to make truly informed decisions about quality further assures that patient decision-making authority is limited.

Healthcare professionals, particularly doctors and nurses who are employees or are acting under contract to the HCO, have their own sets of professional ethical obligations. These independent professional standards, established by professional associations, cannot be controlled by the HCO, but are important factors in the care provided by any HCO. The tension between professional ethical mandates, particularly those that demand that the individual patient always comes first, and contractual obligations to the HCO, which often require attention to the needs of a group of "subscribers" rather than one individual patient, is an ever present source of conflict in today's healthcare organization. At the same time, a HCO cannot function well without excellent professionals. Processes for resolving these tensions need to be fully articulated, developed, and understood by all who are affected by the decisions.

Last, most other institutions providing a social service do so under the auspices of a governmental or charitable agency and do not have to be concerned with the usual market and financial issues which affect all businesses. An HCO, if it is to remain viable and fulfill its mission in today's rapidly changing healthcare arena, must plan for and respond appropriately to marketplace forces, while maintaining a coherent vision of its values and their meaning. Even religious-based HCOs or those who are community-supported must remain economically viable while providing high-quality care in order to survive.

These and other factors bring into question the contention that health care is a commodity or a purely market product. In addition to the division of payers from consumers, the information asymmetry between professionals and patients (and indeed, between healthcare professionals and nonprofessional HCO managers) complicates "customer" relationships since the patient is not the fiscal agent and is almost always vulnerable. There is also a supply/demand asymmetry, since an HCO ordinarily cannot respond to all consumer demands, in particular the demands of the uninsured, without threatening its economic survival. Moreover, some patients or patient groups cannot pay for the health care they need or consume while others pay for more than they consume.

Because HCOs are not ordinary business corporations, Kate Christensen, among others, has argued that all healthcare organizations should be not-for-profit (Christensen, 1996). This position seems both unrealistic and unnecessary. It is unrealistic because there has been a massive conversion in the last fifteen years of nonprofit HMOs to for-profit HMOs (in 1981, 82 percent of HMOs were nonprofit; in 1995, 71 percent of HMOs were for-profit—Isaacs, Beatrice, & Carr 1997, p. 228). It is unnecessary because the market asymmetries and scarcity of resources, both of which affect health care, have similar effects on both for-profit and nonprofit HCOs, creating economic pressures and dilemmas as to how to provide care, how much care to provide, and to whom. We argue in Chapter 4 that attention to profitability is not a problem in itself. It is only problematic if profit-maximizing activities are given priority over activities that maintain a high quality of patient care. It is the priority of values that differentiates organizations—not their nonprofit or for-profit status. In an excellent healthcare organization the actitities and decisions of the HCO reveal patient care to be its highest priority.

ORGANIZATION ETHICS: INTEGRATION OF PATIENT CARE ETHICS, BUSINESS ETHICS, AND PROFESSIONAL ETHICS

If an HCO is to develop a meaningful organization ethics program with adequate mechanisms to deal with the ethical problems it will necessarily encounter, it must develop mechanisms that support the differing ethical perspectives of patient care (clinical) ethics, business ethics, and professional ethics that enable each to enhance the overall ethics program. Organization ethics must work to integrate these perspectives into a unified organization program that promotes and sustains a positive ethical climate within each particular HCO.

Patient care (clinical) ethics

"Rights" movements began in the early sixties with the civil rights movement. Self-determination in a capitalistic democratic society became an acknowledged and undisputed right of the individual. Society looked for ways to protect this right for the disadvantaged and powerless, particularly in research and medical settings. With greater attention to self determination came attention to patient rights and mechanisms to assure their rights as autonomous individuals. By the late 1980s and early 1990s attention to clinical ethics and its focus on the autonomy of the patient was common in HCOs. This attention led to the development in HCOs of institutional ethics committees (IECs), which were seen to be protectors of the autonomy of individual patients. IECs accomplished this goal by educating clinicians and others concerning issues related to patient's rights (truthtelling, confidentiality, decision-making capacity, process of informed consent and refusal, end-of-life decision making, futility issues, and individual access and allocation issues), by instituting a process or processes for consultation on specific patient-care-centered ethical problems, by offering analysis of policies affecting patient rights, and by considering appropriate research and evaluation activities also associated with patient rights issues. Additionally, in recent years, many individual clinical ethics committees have expanded their mission to include acting as the internal conscience of the institution and acting as a bridge between the institution and the community it serves.

The JCAHO played a strong role in the institution of patient care ethics committees in today's HCO. In 1991, the JCAHO in its Patient Rights Standards for the first time required that the institutions it accredited have a "mechanism" to address patient care ethical issues (Joint Commission of Accreditation of Healthcare Organizations, 1992). This led to greater attention to the work of the patient care ethics committee and to its becoming an integral part of the patient care activities of the HCO. Although at various levels of development, essentially all

HCOs today have some type of ethics committee or group to address patient care ethics issues.

By and large, clinical ethics committees have not been asked or even allowed to address organization ethics activities in most HCOs. In fact, most committees have shied away from overt business ethics issues. Some IECs are beginning to undertake the early development of organization ethics activities with varying amounts of authority and outside direction. The Virginia Bioethics Network recently approved a set of organization ethics guidelines that suggest that an expanded and modified patient care ethics committee is the appropriate institutional home for development of the organizational ethics program. We shall discuss this point further in Chapter 9.

To date, few have suggested that a patient care ethics committee can undertake organization ethics development without significant modification of mission, membership, and policies. A much broader perspective than patient rights is required to respond appropriately to organization ethics issues. Whether the patient care ethics committee is the appropriate site for this development is still an open question, but one that must be addressed. However, even if the patient care ethics committee continues to operate separately from organization ethics activities, it must be a part of the development of the organization ethics program since its accepted mission cannot be adequately addressed without considering organization ethics issues, such as determining adequate disclosure of economic factors affecting availability and cost of particular interventions, and conflicts of commitment and interest among healthcare professionals working within the HCO.

Business ethics

The emphasis on business ethics by the AHA in its Organization Ethics Initiative is understandable, and markets play an influential role in health care. But this emphasis is likely to prove to be inadequate, because of the factors emphasized previously: the separation of the payer and the ultimate consumer, the level of knowledge of the ultimate consumer and his insulation from the subtleties of economic decisions concerning healthcare interventions, and the crucial role of professionals in providing services in the HCO, giving priority to economic value-added activities, a priority often (but not always) exhibited in other market-driven organizations, may prove to be damaging to what is in the best interest of the HCO.

Recent work in business ethics has depended heavily on a "stakeholder" concept as the basis for organizational ethical decision making. Under this model, it is the role of those involved to weigh the obligations of the organization to the interested and affected stakeholders, usually believed to include stockholders, customers, payers (if different from customers), employees, contractual partners, the local community, and the larger society.

Critics of the stakeholder concept call attention to its inability to "settle" any-thing, since it is only a framework for developing processes to address specific problems. However, stakeholder theory sees itself as a normative theory that speci-fies reciprocal accountability relationships between stakeholders and the organi-zation in question, and that imports morally relevant standards for evaluating prioritization and decision criteria (Freeman, 1984). There are other problems, however, with using a traditional stakeholder concept to address organization ethics in HCOs. In many other businesses, the role of each stakeholder can be clearly identified. Along with this identification comes mechanisms for each stakeholder (individual or group) to have appropriate decision-making authority in the aspects of the business that affect the stakeholder as a manager or as a part of the organi-zation. This authority is maintained by the assigning of rights and responsibilities based on the particular role. This is made difficult in HCOs because of the con-fusion of roles of the consumer (patient), the buyer or payer (employer, govern-ment, insurance, or managed care organization), the healthcare professional, the manager (who is sometimes a healthcare professional as well), and the HCO itself, which often functions as provider, rationer, and controller of healthcare delivery. If stakeholder theory is to be effective in fostering a positive ethical cli-mate for the organization and developing mechanisms to resolve differences among the groups which comprise the HCO, organization ethics must be able to address not only the often divergent interests of these individuals and groups, but also the role confusion, the markedly different levels of power and authority, and the greater level of social obligation of the HCO. In Chapter 4 we shall present a modified version of stakeholder theory that addresses some, but not all, of these demands.

Professional ethics

The oldest traditional method for considering ethical issues in healthcare has been reliance on and support for the professional ethics of medicine and nursing. Tra-ditional professional ethics is based on the ideal that a healthcare professional should always be an advocate for the particular patient and act in that patient's best interest. There has always been some difficulty with this basic ideal since few, if any, physicians and nurses have been able to act solely for the benefit of one specific patient for any significant length of time. Conflicts with another patient's needs, fiscal demands, and the personal needs of the physician or nurse have always been ethical issues for conscientious physicians and nurses. None-theless, the ideal of advocacy for individual patients has always been, and contin-ues to be, a strong influence on the perceptions and reality of modern healthcare delivery.

Can this traditional professional ideal, articulated and supported in professional codes, be even the beginning of the development of a realistic organization ethics program in a HCO? The answer is obvious. Professional ethics focuses on obligations to specific patients, just as institutional ethics committees focus on the rights of individual patients. An institutional patient care ethics committee may be able to change its mandate, but it is doubtful that a traditional professional ethical perspective would be able to change in such a fundamental way. Professional ethics depends on the character and virtue of the professional for its authority; patient care ethics committees depend on the application of recognized principles related to individual rights for their authority. Neither, as presently constituted, can be the sole basis for organization ethics.

CONCLUSION

Given the limitations of patient care ethics and professional ethics, and the market forces that influence healthcare delivery today, it seems, by default, to leave business ethics and its stakeholder concept as the only possible mechanism to effectively and realistically address the issues of organization ethics. But this is not true. An HCO can appoint an ethics team of administrators, financial officers, business office directors, and others to develop the required organizational code of ethics, and because of their knowledge of administrative and financial issues, this team may perform this task well. This activity will be suspect, however, if it ignores critical aspects of an HCO. An HCO, by definition, is a *healthcare* organization, so its primary mission is to deliver health care to patients or a defined patient population. Every healthcare organization that is a provider organization depends on qualified professionals to deliver that service. In articulating a values statement for all aspects of organizational activity, and in developing a realistic mission statement based on the values statement and the perceived mission of the entire HCO, and lastly in defining a positive ethical climate for all the HCO's staff, employees, professionals, consumers, contractual partners, and community, merely focusing on the "business" aspects of the organization will not accomplish these tasks.

If organization ethics is to have real meaning and the ability to carry out its mandated tasks, it must be based on a mission and a vision of the ethical climate under which the organization defines itself by its ethical values. The organization must then institute processes to ensure that this definition is understood and advanced by all in the organization. This requires supporting patient, business, and professional perspectives when support enhances the organization's ethical climate. But it also requires integrating these three perspectives and mediating among them when integration or mediation is required to advance a positive ethical climate. This will be a difficult task, but its rewards should be many and obvious. How such a task can be accomplished will be outlined in the chapters to follow.

2

A Philosophical Basis for Organization Ethics

Recent upheavals in the way health care is delivered in the United States have called into prominence conflicts between traditional business goals such as efficiency, cost-effectiveness, and productivity, and the ends of such well-established and traditional professions as medicine, nursing, dentistry and the allied health professions. Since many healthcare workers suddenly find themselves playing dual roles as professionals and as employees of healthcare businesses, clashes between competing obligations and responsibilities are rife. The entry of businesses from other areas, such as insurance companies and multinational corporations, into what was traditionally the social welfare arena of health has produced crises, scandals, and increased public scrutiny that have turned health care into one of the most controversial fields of the 1990s.

Many of the most publicized issues have been cases of improper business practices easily analyzed—and prevented—by already available understandings of legal and ethical business dealings. Much less visible are the tensions, frustrations, and conflicts produced within and between people struggling to carry out their traditional obligations responsibly under rapidly changing conditions. Physicians and other healthcare professionals in unprecedented numbers are confronting the problems of maintaining professional integrity in the absence of their traditional autonomy and control over their conditions of practice. They are joining the ranks of engineers, chemists, or meteorologists—countless other professionals, including some healthcare professionals, whose professional codes of ethics, unlike those of the physician, may have been formed under conditions of limited autonomy and constrained choices.

In developing a framework for organization ethics in health care, it would be presumptuous to pretend to begin ex nihilo, and fortunately it is not necessary. The care of the ill has been recognized as a social obligation and a professional responsibility since the beginning of history, and contemporary healthcare organizations are the beneficiary of centuries of tradition and discussion. In particular, the three areas of professional ethics, business ethics, and clinical ethics have extensive literature that can be mined for insights into the problem of establishing an excellent ethical climate in healthcare organizations. In this chapter, we will deal with the philosophical basis for ethics that underlies clinical ethics, business ethics, and professional ethics. In the next three chapters we will examine the ethical resources available to HCOs in those three areas, and suggest reasons why the current state of each of the three applied-ethics areas needs to be supplemented and integrated to meet the needs of contemporary HCOs.

In writing a book on organization ethics, we are presupposing a controversial position: that one can meaningfully use ethical terms to refer not only to individuals, but also to healthcare organizations as well. In ethical terms, for some of the same purposes, we are able to judge between better and worse organizations, to evaluate normatively the actions taken by organizations, their relation to other organizations, and the procedures, practices, and policies that constitute their organizational structure. In the process, we will develop an understanding of what we mean by the "ethical climate" of an organization as a preparation for discussing organization ethics as a procedural approach to initiating or improving the ethical climate.

Although controversial, our approach is not unique. There has been considerable discussion of the moral status of corporations in the literature of business ethics (French, 1979; Goodpaster, 1982; Keeley, 1988; May, 1987; M. Phillips, 1992; Velasquez, 1983; Werhane, 1985). As we saw in Chapter 1, healthcare organizations have some features that distinguish them from most non-healthcare-related business corporations. Still, the analysis of the sense in which the latter may be considered moral agents applies equally to the former. Although constituted for different social purposes than many business corporations and operating under a different legal status, healthcare organizations share enough characteristics with corporations to have a similar moral status. Additionally, because they are in the business of health care, it could be argued that HCOs have even greater obligations to social responsibility than many business corporations. Therefore, it makes sense to consider the HCO as subject to moral judgments.

In what follows we propose a view of the HCO as a moral agent as well as a subject of ethical evaluation, although the moral agency of organizations will not be the same as that of individuals. Organization ethics, as we understand it, is an administratively driven process that is inclusive of, but not exhaustively defined by, the areas of clinical ethics, professional ethics, and business ethics, allowing the HCO and its constituents to better serve its various stakeholders. Organization ethics is the study of institutional moral agency, the analysis of institutional culture, and the explanation of how institutions make decisions that may or may not create a balance of benefits over harms, that respect its members and other institutions, that are or are not fair, or that manifest a good (or questionable) moral character. As a normative activity, organization ethics evaluates and prescribes the kinds of institutional structures that best lend themselves to creating a positive moral climate, a positive ethical culture, within an organization. Organization ethics for HCOs is designed to take into consideration the multiple layers of ethical obligations of the HCO. It examines how HCOs can maximize the ability of the organization to meet them in a way consonant with the professional obligations of its constituent members and the business requirements of the organization, while protecting the clinical arena in which the organization fulfills its primary obligations, which are to the patients and populations that it serves.

WHAT IS ETHICS?

Ethics is defined in a number of overlapping ways. Ethics is the study of what is valued, what is right or wrong, and good or bad, for human beings. The study of ethics (metaethics or theoretical ethics) focuses on the analysis of value, the meaning of terms such as *good* or *right* and the nature of central notions such as choice, freedom, obligation, and responsibility. "Ethics" is a course title in many academic departments, in which case it can be a history of the various ways in which many ethical terms have been defined by traditional figures, or an analytic (metaethical) study of these central notions. The ethical tradition, as studied in philosophy and theology, is a tradition of delineating and defending different answers to questions of value and recommended behavior.

Applied ethics is derived from theoretical ethics. "Conceived broadly, applied ethics is the investigation of the ethical aspects of any problem, personal or social, or any policy or practice. Taken narrowly, applied ethics is the branch of practical reasoning in which ethical reasons, rules, principles, ideals and values are used to evaluate the conduct of individuals or groups" (Bedau, 1992, p. 49). Applied ethics includes traditional casuistry—the application of ethical reflection to cases of practical concern. Applied ethics includes business ethics, clinical ethics, engineering ethics, professional ethics, and legal ethics. If applied ethics is the examination of the role of normative judgments in specific areas of human endeavor, organization ethics itself, as a study of the elements, values, and structures that go into making an organization ethically integrated and responsive, constitutes one type of applied ethics.

Ethics, and thus applied ethics, is also normative: it recommends, prescribes, critiques, and evaluates character, values, practices, and choices, appealing to traditional norms such as utility, respect for persons, fairness, and virtue. It is normatively that ethics is featured in codes of ethics—whether for lawyers, managers, physicians, administrators, or nurses—individuals playing various roles in society or in social institutions. Normative evaluation presupposes that individuals have some degree of freedom of action. They have needs, interests, or desires that serve as motives to action. They seek to attain their objectives by choosing among the courses of action that are available to them; and those objectives themselves are to some extent chosen by them. The three poles of ethical evaluation, then, focus on agents, actions, and outcomes (see Table 2.1). We commend or discourage objectives, encourage or disapprove of alternative means of reaching those objectives, and evaluate the relations of individuals to other particular individuals or to the society in which they live. We speak of the duties owed to other members of the society, or obligations toward them; of the rights of ourselves or of others; and of traits of character, habits, or actions as being morally admirable or reprehensible. Many ethics books take one of these evaluative poles as primary and construct ethical theories which are oriented toward character and intentions (virtue), rules and principles (deontological), or outcomes (consequentialist). Our approach is pluralistic and practice oriented, rather than theory driven, but the distinction between poles of ethical evaluation will be useful in some of our discussion.

Although individuals, as agents, are subject to moral evaluation, the criteria by which they are evaluated do not typically come merely from themselves. The standards by which we evaluate the actions and choices of others are often common to all members of the society and are frequently spelled out in and enforced by legal sanctions as well. They may vary in some respects from society to society, as history and anthropology tell us; or in some details from one religious, ethnic, or social group to another within the same society. Within varyingly broad or narrow limits, these divergences are themselves tolerated or sanctioned in different ways in different societies. The amount of deviation from acceptable standards that is tolerated, and the mechanisms of reward or sanction, are defining characteristics not only of societies, but of various subgroups within societies.

TABLE 2.1. Poles of Ethical Evaluation

AGENTS	ACTIONS	OUTCOMES
Character	Right/wrong	Objectives
Motives/intentions	Duties/obligations	Consequences
Consistency	Legal/illegal	Intended or unintended

One sometimes appeals to what are contended to be universal or absolute values, standards that are, or should be, applicable to all individuals and societies everywhere. The notorious difficulty is, of course, that philosophers cannot agree on what these standards are or should be, and examinations of the great religions gives evidence that there are both congruencies and differences in what absolute standards should be. Still, it is true that in making moral evaluations we appeal to standards that we claim should be cross-cultural or universal. This is part of making moral judgments. So the process of moral evaluation includes an ongoing process of proposing and challenging standards of judgment even though we may not reach agreement nor ever be able to verify which standards are indeed absolute ones.

Michael Walzer has proposed an interesting way to think about universal values. Walzer argues that throughout history and in different cultures there is a thin thread of coherence and agreement. The agreement is less about what is *good*, but rather on some at least partial universal recognition of "bads." For example, Walzer argues that while there is wide disagreement about definitions or theories of justice, there is mutual recognition of *injustice*. We are uncertain about the constitution of the "good life," but there is widespread agreement about deficient or despicable living conditions, indecencies, violations of human rights, mistreatment, and other harms. We are all in agreement that Bhopal and *Challenger* were disasters. We are less certain about how to prevent such future disasters. We concur that the healthcare system in the United States is in difficulty. But we cannot agree on solutions. These moral minimums, what we agree are *bads*, are best understood as negative standards, universally agreed upon "bottom lines" beyond which it is morally questionable to act. For example, it is almost always wrong to deliberately harm or contribute to harming another person or persons, to deliberately violate their rights to freedom, life, or property, to treat individuals or classes of individuals with disrespect, to compete or cooperate unfairly, not to honor promises or contract, or to be dishonest or deceitful. These moral minimums do not spell out what goodness, fairness, or benefit is. Neither do they spell out the positive content of rights. They do, however, set minimum guidelines for behavior that most people everywhere might agree on. A basis for common-sense morality, and the notion of moral minimums, gives a strong counterargument to those who find values as merely context dependent (Walzer, 1994; Werhane, 1998b).

Ethics is also descriptive, and as such it depends upon its normative role. Anthropology, sociology, management studies, social psychology, and foreign policy, among others, study differences in ways of life and rules of conduct in different groups, differences in moral codes, the way people acquire moral values, and the impact of different social structures on morality. Professional journals of nursing, medicine, and business are filled with studies of how various individuals and groups make ethical decisions, factors that influence choices, and descriptions of human relationships, culture, practices, and levels of evaluation.

THE SUBJECT MATTER FOR ETHICS AND APPLIED ETHICS

Traditionally, ethics has focused on the study, prescription, evaluation and description of the motivation, choices, values, character, and actions of individual human beings. Despite this preoccupation with the individual and with individual behavior, one must always be reminded that human beings are social beings. Who we are and how we develop depends on the social, historical, and political context in which we find ourselves and interact, as even the Enlightenment philosopher Adam Smith argued (Smith, 1976). This is not to argue that we are *determined* by the community in which we grow up, but who we are and how we think about moral issues develops out of and is never completely independent of the social context and historical conditions in which we become adults.

Therefore, it is not strange that moral terms such as *right* and *wrong* are used to evaluate institutional and social decisions and outcomes as well. We hold institutions and even social systems as well as individuals morally responsible. In applied ethics, moral terms such as *right* and *wrong*, *good* and *evil* are also used to analyze, evaluate, and describe motivations, practices, and outcomes of larger social units: institutions, organizations, and even political units. Ethical considerations can be invoked on three levels: the individual, or microethical level, scrutinizing choices and characters of persons; on the organizational level, involving policies and cultures of organizations and institutions; and on the macroethical, or political, level, where we can apply moral criteria such as justice and degree of

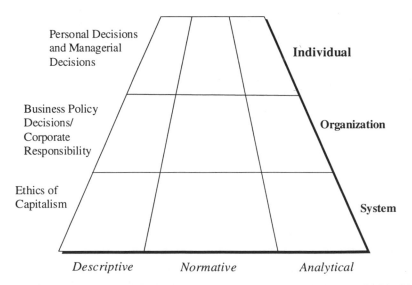

FIGURE 2.1. Wide and narrow issues in business ethics related to divisions of ethical inquiry. From Goodpaster, 1984, p. 296.

participation in decision making to the arrangements and ideologies of entire social systems (Goodpaster, 1984).

In this book we will concentrate our attention on organizations, and we will
focus primarily on normative elements of institutional-level ethics in healthcare
organizations. In focusing on the midlevel agency, organizations, it is necessary
to acknowledge that the agency, actions, and effects of organizational decision
making have implications for both other levels. The society of which HCOs are a
part has expectations of the function of the HCO which are tacit as well as explicit, and enforced, however efficiently, by rewards and sanctions, both moral
and legal. The persons who constitute the HCO or are immediately affected by its
actions also have justified expectations and judge the organization to be good or
bad, a moral or immoral agent in all its poles of evaluation.

We choose to focus on the ethics of the middle level because of our conviction
that this is both effective and appropriate. We assume that "the values of the or
ganization are not a simple or straightforward function of either the values of the
surrounding system or the values of the individuals in the organization" (Goodpaster, 1992, p. 112). As we focus on the policies and culture of the HCO, we do
so in a way that acknowledges the implication of those factors on the choices and
character of the individuals implicated in the operations of the HCO.

FORMAL ORGANIZATIONS, BUREAUCRACIES, AND OPEN SYSTEMS

Organization ethics focuses on the ethical dimensions of midlevel phenomena:
organizations: their motives, the nature and quality of their actions, and the effects
of their actions. One possibility in thinking about the ethics of healthcare organizations is to appeal to the literature on formal organizations or bureaucracies.
Organizations, particularly large organizations, often function as bureaucracies
or as "formal organizations." A formal organization is an impersonal "decision-
making structure" (Simon, 1965, p. 9) where choices of the organization are
executed in terms of its mission, goals, and culture. Organizational decisions are
social decisions made by individuals on behalf of the organization, and the
decisions are attributable to the organization rather than to the individual organizational decision maker. According to proponents of organizational theory, a well-
functioning formal organization is one that achieves its ends efficiently and thoroughly with the fewest possible side effects or externalities.

Because formal organizational decision making is done by individuals or groups
of individuals acting on behalf of the organization (Ladd, 1970, p. 501), each individual in the organization has a defined role, and in theory, at least, the role
decisions are impersonal choices made from the perspective of the organization,
its purpose and mission. Each individual, while working in the formal organiza-

tion, is a placeholder who is expected to carry out her role obligations in her official capacity as defined by the organization, rather than consider her own interests, values, or professional commitments. Bureaucratic ethics, under the rubric of formal organizations, evaluates an organization and organizational decision making in terms of an "ideal of rationality," defined as how well organizational ends are achieved by its placeholder decisions and actions. Thus a rational decision is one that is "efficient in pursuing a desired goal, whatever it may be" (Ladd, 1970; Scott, 1998).

In the first instance, then, a formal organization is evaluated in terms of how well it achieves its mission and goals. However, if understood literally as a closed system, so-called bureaucratic ethics appears to conflate rationality with morality. Sometimes we conclude that a well-run organization is a good, morally good, organization. One sees examples—the Mafia is one—of organizations where each constituent achieved his role obligations and the organization ran efficiently to achieve its ends. Yet because of its activities, the organization would be questionable from a moral point of view. One could also imagine the converse, for example, a HCO whose primary and stated mission was profitability. Yet its activities efficiently and effectively provided good-quality health care to a defined population.

One could also envision an organization, whose mission and aims were exemplary, yet the means to produce those aims might entail consequences that are morally questionable. For example, a military organization's mission might be to defend the nation, usually a worthwhile aim. Still, we need to evaluate the structure of that organization to see whether the means to achieve that mission encourage violations of human rights, misuse of power, or other untoward activities. Similarly, an HCO whose mission was patient or population health has the promise of a good organization. Still, we need to evaluate the means that each HCO uses to achieve that noble end.

Thus, while bureaucratic ethics describes ways in which organizations act as impersonal agents and prescribe role obligations, we also judge the moral worth of an organization in terms of its mission, structure, culture, activities, and what those activities produce or fail to achieve. These sorts of judgments can only be executed by stepping back from the organization and appealing to more general principles, and by reflecting, as well, upon the relationships the organization has with other levels depicted in Figure 2.1. Properly conceived, then, organization ethics requires appeals outside the bureaucracy or organization in question to judge both (1) whether the organization and its mission are justified and (2) whether what the organization justifies or produces is morally acceptable (Luben, 1988, pp. 133–134).

In a recent article, Allen Buchanan tries to develop a theory of bureaucratic ethics that appeals to principal/agent risk. Buchanan defines a bureaucratic organization as "a complex web of principal/agent relationships" (Buchanan, 1996, p. 424), where "agents" are persons who are engaged to perform tasks on behalf of the organization as directed by the "principals" or top management. Ethical principles "include principles that express commitments that function as internal constraints on agents to reduce risks to the legitimate interests of principals" (ibid.). Buchanan avoids the difficulty of evaluating an organization on grounds other than its own mission, defined relationships, and agent commitment by introducing an important role for ethical principles to evaluate both the placeholder roles of agents and the organization itself. The difficulty with Buchanan's proposal is unpacking the notion of principal/agent relationships in ways that illustrate the complexity of these relationships in HCOs. Moreover, unless principal/agent relationships are redefined adequately, these relationships will not accurately depict the maze of overlapping relationships between professionals, managers, organizations, and patient care.

Karl Weick raises questions about reifying organizations. "The word, organization, is a noun and it is also a myth. If one looks for an organization one will not find it. What will be found is that there are events, linked together, that transpire within concrete walls and these sequences, their pathways, their timing, are the forms we erroneously make into substances when we talk about an organization" (Weick, 1974, p. 358). According to Weick, a more fruitful way, which is particularly suited to HCOs, is to think of organizations, as open systems. Organizations, according to this view, are best thought of as systems that are created by, and interact with, changing sets of agents and within a dynamic social environment in which they find themselves. Organizations are made up of a complex of changing, dynamic interrelationships through which the organization defines and regenerates itself and even metamorphoses as it interacts with changing surroundings. This way of thinking about organizations accounts for change, as illustrated in the dramatic changes in healthcare organizations in the last twenty years, and it gives credence to the idea that organizations, like people, are subject to moral judgments that are not merely internally self-referential.

ROLES AND ROLE MORALITY

There is another set of reasons why the ethics of closed formal organizations or bureaucratic ethics is a flawed model. Social institutions, including organizations, can enhance or impair the moral agency of individuals employed by them, by the structural integration of the elements of the institution itself. Institutions are normatively judged on the extent to which they accommodate the moral agency of the individuals whose activities constitute the organization. Thus a thorough organization ethics for HCOs must focus not merely on the ethical issues facing the organization and individuals within the organization. It must also analyze roles and role morality, and reciprocal moral relationships and responsibilities between institutions and individuals. "'Role' refer[s] to constellations of institutionally specified rights and duties organized around an institutionally specified social function . . . [where] 'an institution [is any public system or social arrangement that] includes rules that define offices and positions which can be occupied by different individuals at different times'" (Hardimon, 1994, pp. 334–335). There are a set of impersonal socially defined collections of expectations and demands that comes with each role, and when we take on a role we assume certain rights and duties. In addition, most roles are usually associated with ideals, norms that define, for example, the perfect mother or the ideal firefighter (Downie, 1971; Emmet, 1966; Hardimon, 1994; Luben, 1988; Werhane, 1985; 1998a). Thus along with each role are moral demands spelled out by that role, and these define what is called "role morality" (Luben, 1988; Andre, 1991).

Role morality describes and evaluates the extent to which one succeeds in meeting the demands and obligations of one's role. Role morality in organizations describes and evaluates accountability relationships between an organization and its constituents, and judges whether an individual placeholder has fulfilled her obligations as defined by her roles. In bureaucracies, and elsewhere, one is expected to "do one's duties" as defined by the organization, and ordinarily there are good moral reasons for acting according to role demands. Indeed, if people did not do so most of the time, social relationships and organizational activities would be chaotic. As Judith Andre has carefully argued, the existence of roles and role obligations permits a predictability of human behavior and a stability in social relationships. Both a mother who ignores her children and a manager who does not take seriously his fiduciary responsibilities to his company are, under most circumstances, judged to be immoral by the standards of role morality and by the judgment of any commonsense perspective. The well-being of any organization depends on the fulfillment of role obligations by its constituents (Andre, 1991).

However, and this is where bureaucratic ethics falls short in closed systems, role morality is not sufficiently able to evaluate constituent behavior. If organizational structures and climate mandate questionable activities, as might be possible in some organizations, one needs to be able to evaluate roles, role obligations, and role acts not merely in terms of the organizational mission but also in more general terms of commonsense morality. One could imagine an HCO with an appropriate mission to safeguard the health of its patients or of a particular targeted population. Yet one could also imagine that within that organization the admissions staff is not allowed to accept new patients who are HIV infected. Healthcare professionals within this organization are given limits for costs of prescriptions that will exclude HIV infected patients from being eligible for the AIDS "cocktail." In this case, the healthcare professional's role as a professional clashes with her role expectations and obligations as an employee. On a more dramatic level, we often judge someone negatively *because* of the role obligations they performed. Those in Nazi Germany, and more recently the Hutus in Rwanda, who obeyed orders and performed their assigned roles well, are condemned precisely because they exemplified perfect role morality (Arendt, 1963).

Because as human beings we are not exhaustively defined by our roles, each of us can stand apart from and evaluate our roles and role responsibilities. We can and should use those same tools of common morality for judging roles and role obligations that we use for evaluating organizations. Just as we evaluate and assess organizations and institutions, we can also evaluate organizationally defined roles and the ends they allegedly serve. Part of organization ethics is the evaluation of any role, its role-defined obligations, the organization to which it is attached, and whatever acts the role, role duties, and organization seem to demand. We also evaluate the role, role obligations, as well as the organization or institution as to what the organization, role, obligation, or act justifies in the form of organizational activities (Luben, 1988, Chapters 6 and 7).

THE MORAL STATUS OF ORGANIZATIONS

An organization is neither an individual nor a total social system. It is a subunit of the larger society, comprising individuals in various roles and authorized by the larger society to function for specific, often narrowly defined, purposes. Thus an organization such as an HCO has ethical orientations in several directions: toward the society of which it is a component; toward other institutions, organizations or corporations with which it interrelates; and toward individuals: both those individuals who constitute the organization, its members, and toward the individuals and populations served by, and serving, the organization as well.

Laws govern many organizational relationships on every level. The charter of an HCO, for example, gives it certain legal privileges in exchange for its commitment to deliver health care to the community in which it is located. Contracts between the HCO and its suppliers of equipment, services, or pharmaceuticals are subject to the laws that cover contracts in the larger society, as are many aspects of employee relations. HCOs that are incorporated, like business corporations, are treated as legal persons under the law and are granted many of the same constitutional rights as individuals. But the relation of law and ethics is far from simple. Although HCOs, like other organizations, are of course expected to operate within the limits of the law, that does not exhaust their ethical obligations. They have obligations in many areas in which the law is silent. Moreover, recognition under the law and/or legal personhood does not translate into moral personhood. Still, although organizations are not individuals, and therefore are not moral persons, they can be meaningfully said to be moral agents in several senses.

1. Organizations, like individuals, set goals. These goals are often specified in mission statements, delineated in charters, or defined by the founding arrangements that constitute the organization as a corporate entity.
2. Organizations "act," although the actions of an organization are often the result of collective, not individual, decision making. The policies of an organization arise from deliberation between possible courses of action to meet organizational goals. Courses of organizational action are selected that involve both their external constituencies (payers, suppliers, government agencies, and contracting organizations) and their internal constituencies (employees, stockholders, associated professionals, served patients and populations).
3. Organizations, as well as individuals, are normatively evaluated. They are judged to be morally acceptable or unacceptable by other organizations with which they interact, by the individuals who come in contact with them either as constituent members or as recipients of their services, and also by the larger society, which has entrusted the organization with certain social responsibilities. Just as individuals are expected to meet their responsibilities and are blamed if they fail to do so, corporations and other organizations have responsibilities and are expected to meet them.
4 Organizations are held accountable on all the poles of normative evaluation: as agents, on the nature of their actions, and by the effects of their actions. They meet—or fail to meet—expectations, and are subject to praise or blame on the basis of their achievements. Organizations are judged good or bad, excellent or immoral, on various criteria: on how well they treat the individuals who collectively constitute the organization; on how well their decisions and policies satisfy the interests and objectives of the various individuals or groups who have a stake in the organization; on how well the organization fulfills its mission, both as stated in its own goals, and as understood by the larger society in which it plays a role; and on whether the actions of the organization fall within the ethical and legal prescriptions of the larger society of which it is a component.

Because organizations have many of the characteristics of individual human moral agents, it is tempting to argue that organizations are identical to moral persons, at least to the extent that they are full-fledged moral agents (French, 1979). But this theory, while of theoretical interest, takes us too far afield. Organizations do not literally act; they cannot. Their actions ultimately depend on decisions and actions of individuals. Moreover, to claim that organizations are full-fledged moral agents intimates that they have the status of individual moral agents. But since they cannot make choices or act, except collectively, this is a very strange conclusion. Moreover, while we hold organizations morally accountable, we do not, on this account, want to let individuals working in and for organizations off the hook. Because organizations and organizational actions are a result of human creativity and choice, individuals, too, are accountable for organizational action.

On the other hand, organizations, at least medium-sized and large organizations, function as systems, so one cannot treat organizations merely as aggregates, considering ethical issues of organizations to be reducible to or discussed only in terms of the ethical issues faced by the individuals who severally constitute those organizations (Velasquez, 1983). To try to reduce all organizational motives, processes, behavior, and outcomes to individual motives, actions, and consequences, cannot adequately account for organizational action. Organizations do have a purpose for being; they often have mission statements, credos, or other statements of purpose that set the framework for organizational decision making. They set and change goals, and those working within or for the organization act with those purposes, statements, and goals in mind. It is true that the purposes, mission, and goals of any organization are created by groups of individuals; nevertheless, these phenomena function as guides for individual and group organizational behavior, *as if* the organization was an individual directing the activities of its constituents.

Group dynamics of those acting on behalf of the organization are such that many actions of an organization are collective actions in another sense. Individuals and groups within organizations act as agents for organization, deriving their direction from its mission and goals. As a result, many actions or sets of actions are not traceable to, or redescribable in terms of, any one set of individuals who initiated the action. So it is often difficult to hold specific individuals morally responsible for all organizational activities, even though the actions in question were initiated, processed, and carried out by individuals carrying out organizational goals created by individuals. Thus we want to say that organizations are moral agents, and they, like individuals, can be held morally accountable, although they are not identical to individual moral agents, because they do not literally have motives, they do not literally make choices or act (Werhane, 1985).

Organizations are different from individuals in another dimension. Altogether, mission, goals, and constituent collective activities create an organizational culture. E. Jacques (1951) defined *organizational culture* as "[t]he customary or traditional ways of thinking and doing things, which are *shared* to a greater or lesser extent by all members of the organization and which new members of the organization must *learn* and at least partially accept in order to be accepted into the service of the firm" (Jacques, 1951, p. 166).

One component of the organizational culture is what some organizational theorists call the "ethical climate" of an organization. The ethical climate of an organization is the functional analogue of the character of an individual. A person's character is a group of relatively stable traits connected with practical choice and action. Similarly, an organization's ethical climate is defined by the shared perceptions of how ethical issues should be addressed and what is ethically correct behavior for the organization (Victor & Cullen, 1988). Just as personal character often affects what an individual will do when faced with moral dilemmas, corporate ethical climate guides what an organization and its constituents will do when faced with issues of conflicting values. Ethical climate includes both content—the shared perceptions of what constitutes ethical behavior—and process: how ethical issues will be dealt with. In our understanding of organization ethics, the organization ethics processes within an organization such as an HCO are the custodians of the ethical climate, the analogue, on the organizational level, of conscience in an individual.

As used in this chapter, *ethical climate* refers to the character of the organization. There is another usage for this term as well, which we will use in Chapter 7, by which ethical climate refers to the social/political/economic/religious environment in which an individual or an organization is embedded. In this usage it is obvious that the external ethical climate can affect the organization and its internal climate. These effects are important to recognize as part of the causes for the rapid changes in healthcare organizations in the 1990s. More will be said about these influences in Chapters 6 and 7.

ORGANIZATIONAL EVALUATION AND ETHICAL THEORY

Part of organization ethics is the moral evaluation of the organization itself: its mission, culture, climate, and activities; another part is the moral evaluation of organizational roles and role obligations, and those activities mandated by role obligations. We must now consider the kinds of criteria appropriate to such evaluations. As we noted earlier, ethical theorists often choose one of the evaluative poles of agent, action, or outcome as primary. They then construct ethical theories that give priority to one of these poles and evaluate the morality of their object according to that standard. In applied ethics this same tendency can be observed.

Some philosophers equate good organizational decision making with character and virtue, arguing that the best managers and professionals and best organizations exhibit the civic virtues of integrity, good judgment, community spirit, honor, loyalty, or even a sense of shame (Solomon, 1992). Thus organizations, like individuals, can be judged to have or lack good character. Part of organizational character is reflected in its culture and climate as well as in the day-to-day activities of the organization. The development of good constituent and organizational corporate moral character is essential, it is argued, for organizational good citizenship, to prevent harms and violations of rights, and to promote the long-term well-being of the organization and its stakeholders (Solomon, 1992).

Other thinkers in applied ethics use more consequentialist tests for the moral value of the decision or action in question. Since much of applied decision making is a matter of weighing costs versus benefits, a consequentialist or utilitarian approach makes sense in evaluating the ethical dimensions of a decision as well. From this approach it is often argued that evaluating decisions should be a process of weighing benefits against harms. An action that on balance contributes negatively to the organization, is unprofitable, or harms its stakeholders or the community, all things considered, is at best a questionable action (Bentham, 1948).

A more deontological or rules-based approach would argue that a goal, a decision, or action that uses people as means for other objectives would be one that would not meet this moral criterion. Respect for autonomy and rights trump other concerns. In addition to autonomy and respect for individuals, procedural fairness, informed consent, contractual agreements, exit and governance are means tests for roles and role obligations (Kant, 1956; Bowie, 1999).

From a justice perspective, one might argue that organizations, like individuals, are required to meet the moral requirements of equity, consistency, and impartiality. So a process or procedure that does not offer equal opportunity, that judges persons or institutions on irrelevant criteria, that does not reward equitably, that overcharges or misinforms its customers, violates contractual agreements, or that in other respects is unfair to any or to some stakeholders, is questionable from a moral point of view (Velasquez, 1998).

A more general approach would be to begin with Walzer's notion of moral minimums. Commonly held minimum standards are those shared commitments to what most, if not all, would agree are the "bads." They include gratuitous harm, unfair practices, processes, or outcomes; lying; breaking promises and contracts; and not respecting individuals and their rights. Tools for evaluation include appeals to the precepts of common morality, those rules or precepts that most of us, stepping out of our roles and judging others, would regard as rules for how we and others ought to behave (moral rules such as mutual respect, avoidance of harm, respect for rights and fairness, honoring promises and contracts, and respect for property). So actions that on balance create more harm than good or whose costs are greater than their benefits are, at best, questionable actions. Processes and outcomes that treat people unfairly, negate equal opportunity, or violate rights are surely morally unfit. Finally if a practice is one that would be unacceptable in some other context, e.g., most instances of lying or bribery, it is subject to question in organizations as well.

All of these approaches have their limitations; none fits every moral situation. As we noted above, our approach in this book is pluralistic and practice oriented. Rather than adopting a theoretical approach that we then apply to the evaluation of healthcare organizations, we have chosen to start from the standpoint of the organization, invoking various evaluative foci as are relevant. Each evaluative focus is based on the assumption that one can step back from a particular situation or context and make disinterested moral judgments of oneself, of one's roles and role obligations, and of organizations, their mission, culture, and direction. These judgments are not infallible, and we have not yet perfected one theoretical moral model on which to ground our judgments. This pragmatic approach considers moral theories as possible candidates for a model, candidates that we apply contextually and contingently, but nevertheless with some confidence in their general if not universal applicability.

In developing organization ethics, such disinterested judgments and appeals to general moral standards or commonsense morality are essential. From a moral point of view no organization or institution is morally self-contained. Organizations, like people, are fallible and must be continually scrutinized both by their constituents and by outsiders. The limits of bureaucratic ethics and role morality make this clear. Organization ethics requires evaluations of the organization and its constituents, and it requires that these evaluations appeal to standards, minimums, or principles independent of the organization or bureaucracy.

We will consider the strengths and weaknesses of several ethics models in the next chapters. As we shall see, traditional ethical theory is only partly effective in dealing with the ethics of HCOs. Rules and principles are of themselves sometimes both too vague and too narrow to provide effective ethical guidance in problematic situations, specific contexts, and particular kinds of organizations. The approach we take in this book embodies several assumptions about both organizations and the individuals who constitute them that require us to look carefully at the special features of HCOs. HCOs share characteristics with other organizations, but have their own distinct features. HCOs are made up of healthcare professionals, managers, and other employees. They are responsible for patient and population health care, they have obligations to the healthcare insurers who ordinarily are not the patients themselves, and they have duties to the communities in which they operate and serve. To be effective, organization ethics for HCOs must encompass a number of ethical perspectives, allowing and encouraging business, professional, and clinical imperatives to maintain their traditional stances when they can contribute positively to the ethical climate of the HCO. Moreover, organization ethics must focus on the particular ethical issues of institutional practice within each specific organization, and address each with processes for resolution and adjudication, instead of providing prepackaged, one-size fits-all "answers." Different organizations will need to develop appropriate modes of articulating and maintaining the ethical climate of their type of institution. In the next chapters, we will consider these points in more detail.

3

Clinical Ethics and Organization Ethics

It is in the clinical units that the fundamental work of an HCO occurs. However extensive the administrative and support system which grows up around those units, it is here that the excellence or inadequacies of the HCO are most often judged by HCO stakeholders, including patients, staff, and the larger society. The ethics of the clinical enterprise has received a great deal of attention in the last few decades. The public is increasingly aware of ethical issues in health care, and medical innovations constantly force us to rethink issues that seemed settled only yesterday. The shift from individual to team medicine has changed the parameters within which we think of ethical issues in clinical practice, and institutional ethics committees (IECs) have developed as the forum in which competing values are negotiated between team members, or between the medical team and families.

The clinical setting will not decline in importance as a focus for ethical activity in HCOs, but the interpenetration of organizational and clinical ethical decisions is becoming increasingly obvious. All clinical decisions have organizational implications, and the converse is often the case as well. Cases brought to IECs frequently focus on organizational problems that created them, and organizational changes are sometimes suggested in order that the same problem not recur. This tendency has been accelerated by the recent addition of "organization" ethics standards to the JCAHO accreditation procedure and by initiatives from other directions as well. The first response to a request for examples of implementation of these accreditation standards is often to report upon the organizational changes that were recommended in the process of addressing an individual patient care problem.*

In this chapter we will briefly define clinical ethics and look at some of its theoretical and historical underpinnings, as well as the problems it considers in its contemporary practice in the HCO. We complete the chapter with a discussion of clinical ethics' present and future relation to organization ethics.

WHAT IS CLINICAL ETHICS?

Clinical ethics is concerned with the ethics of the clinical practice of medicine and with ethical problems that arise in the care of patients. Ethical perspectives to which it is most closely related include traditional professional medical ethics, theoretical bioethics, and critical social theory. Each of these perspectives has had significant influence on the development of clinical ethics and on its activities and status in today's healthcare system.

Out of attention to deficiencies in traditional medical ethics in the last half of the twentieth century, a broader field, bioethics, emerged. Bioethics' first concern was with "the intersection of ethics and the life sciences" (Callahan, 1995, p. 248), or more generally, with the intersection of life sciences and human values. But bioethics has expanded into an interdisciplinary field concerned with public health, health policies, law, and social issues as these areas affect science, medicine, and ethics. Clinical ethics, in turn, began as a distinct subfield of bioethics because of a perceived need for closer attention to ethical issues associated with specific clinical practices at the bedside, in particular to assure that the rights of the patient be a primary determinate of the direction of medical care. This focus of clinical ethics involves examining individual clinical cases within the context of the institutional and social setting (Siegler, Pellegrino & Singer, 1990). In fulfilling this focus, clinical ethics has relied on a major traditional tenet of professional medical ethics for its primary guidance; that is, it has put care of the individual patient as the first priority in clinical practice.

---

*JCAHO accreditation reviews now ask what institutions are doing about the organizational ethics standard. Informal conversations with ethics committee members from around the country suggest that many of them are explicitly directing their attention to organizational implications of individual case consultations, with very positive results. A typical response: "We addressed the issue of a disruptive patient in one of our facilities. In the process of our research, we found that the sensory environment can strongly affect patient behavior. In addition to our other suggestions, we recommended that the color of the walls in the facility be changed." Clinical ethics at its best has always asked what could have been done to prevent the problem from arising in the first place; but the range of things open to consideration is expanding under the impact of the new standards.

Contemporary clinical ethics has focused almost exclusively on the individual patient and his personal autonomy, not on the larger community. Through IECs it has established itself as an important adjunct to clinical decision making within the HCO. Although the clinical ethics literature does to some extent consider problems that arise in private practice, the main focus has been on problems that arise in institutional settings, reinforcing the HCO as the institutional base for clinical ethics.

Clinical ethics supports a number of well-established avenues to address ethical issues in clinical practice, including IECs found in most HCOs, and ethics networks that function mainly as sources for practical ethics education for specific groups or for a specified geographic area. Solitary consultants or groups of consultants who function as clinical ethics advisors to patients, patients' families, and clinicians, may be employed by HCOs as part of their clinical ethics programs.

Clinical ethics, as it has developed, has tended to use the language of bioethics and has looked to law, public policy, social work, and other social phenomena that influence the emerging complexity of health care to expand its knowledge base for evaluating clinical practices. The priorities, as well as the language, of bioethics inform clinical ethics. However, practitioners of clinical ethics are most often health professionals who have familiarized themselves with the language and issues of bioethics or, in some cases, nonclinicians, including academically-trained bioethicists, who have familiarized themselves with the clinical setting and concentrated on the problems that arise there (Fletcher & Brody, 1995, p. 400).

CLINICAL ETHICS AND TRADITIONAL PROFESSIONAL MEDICAL PRACTICE

Clinical ethics is closely related to professional medical ethics, and shares its governing ideal of attention to the care of the individual patient. It differs significantly from professional medical ethics in being explicitly multidisciplinary, in focusing on the rights of the patient in contrast to the obligations of the physician, and in taking into consideration the contemporary reality of team care in the modern HCO, which integrates practitioners from a variety of different professions.

The ethics of professional medical practice, traditionally a Hippocratic-based physician ethic, is still today one of the important ethical perspectives informing those who care for patients. Nurses and other professionals, including respiratory therapists, chaplains, social workers, and people trained in many other allied health professions, may also be constrained in their role in clinical practice by codes of their specific professions, codes that place differing emphases on one or another of the various values held in common by those codes. Clinical ethics acknowledges that there are important differing professional perspectives involved in clinical practice, and self-consciously tries to compensate for differentials of power among them. The IEC, as clinical ethics' functional mechanism within a HCO, can be a forum for discussion of differences of ethical judgment among members of clinical teams.

THEORETICAL BIOETHICS AND ETHICAL THEORY

Bioethics, as described in the latest edition of the *Encyclopedia of Bioethics*, has several different areas of concern: theoretical, clinical, regulatory/policy, and cultural (Callahan, 1995, pp. 245–256). From this broader standpoint, clinical ethics is indeed, as James F. Childress has said, "a bridge between the world of bioethics and medical humanities and the world of clinicians and patients" (Fletcher, Lombardo, Marshall & Miller, 1995, viii), a component of a wider field. From the standpoint of clinical ethics, on the other hand, bioethics is but one participant in the discussion, along with professional ethics, social expectations, legal strictures, and organizational constraints.

Some theoretical approaches in bioethics are more closely analogous to clinical thinking than others or are more readily adaptable to that context. A number of academic thinkers have specifically concerned themselves with ethical questions arising in the clinical setting and thus have advanced the discourse. They have come from differing theoretical perspectives and applied these perspectives to ethical issues associated with the clinical setting and thereby advanced the theoretical basis for clinical ethics. If a true theory of clinical ethics develops, it is likely to be the product of these academic bioethicists who have the interest and time to develop it. To date, however, clinical ethics itself has been less interested in developing a comprehensive theory, or in deciding between competing ethical theories, than in developing methods for dispute resolution in clinical cases.

Figure 3.1 shows the levels of ethical abstraction, from the most abstract level of ethical theory to the concrete and particular level of the individual problematic clinical case. As we have suggested, clinical ethics starts from and focuses attention on the individual problematic case, and typically moves only as far up the levels of ethical abstraction as is useful in treating the case in question. Thus, although there have been numerous candidate theories proposed for clinical ethics, the most popular approaches, principlism and casuistry, are pluralistic or neutral with respect to general theories of ethics, and concentrate on more concrete levels of discourse.* Because of the practitioner focus and the persistent influence of professional ethics, virtue and character approaches have remained influential among clinical ethicists, and contemporary movements in academic ethics like

---

*Albert Jonsen gives an excellent summary of early work on a general theory of bioethics in Chapter 10 of his 1998 book on the birth of bioethics (Jonsen, 1998).

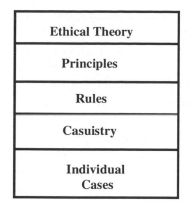

FIGURE 3.1. Levels of ethical abstraction.

feminist ethics of care or clinical pragmatism have had their impact as well. We discuss these theoretical approaches below.

Principlism

One approach that has been extremely fruitful has been termed "principlism" by its adherents and critics alike. In their influential book, *Principles of Biomedical Ethics*, first published in 1979 and now in its fourth edition, Tom L. Beauchamp and James F. Childress articulate and defend an approach that is grounded in common morality (common moral sense and shared tradition) and uses moral principles as its framework. The four principles of respect for autonomy, non-maleficence, beneficence, and justice are proposed as a basic minimum of morally relevant considerations for people who might otherwise disagree about their theoretical foundations. These four principles, if specified in a particular situation and balanced as appropriate, often serve as sufficient common ground to allow for agreement. Similar principles (respect for persons, beneficence, and justice) were articulated as guidelines for federal research in the National Commission for the Protection of Human Subjects of Biomedical and Behavioral Research in 1978.*

Principles, though central to Beauchamp and Childress's position, do not (and should not) provide precise or specific guidelines for every set of circumstances. They require judgment for their application and balance, which in turn depends

---

*The National Commission for the Protection of Human subjects of Biomedical and Behavioral Research, 1978. The commission's general principles appear in *The Belmont Report: Ethical Guidelines for the protection of Human Subjects,* Washington, DC: DHEW Publication (OS) 78–0012, 1978.

upon character, moral discernment, individual responsibility, and accountability (Beauchamp & Childress, 1994, p. 462). Indeed, as Beauchamp and Childress note, many different theories lead to similar action-guides; it is possible from several standpoints to defend roughly the same principles, obligations, rights, responsibilities, and virtues (p. 110). Other analogous approaches appeal to a plurality of rules, often hierarchically ordered (Veatch, 1981; Clouser & Gert, 1990). Principles appealed to by other authors include integrity, honesty, keeping contracts, truth telling, and various (sometimes competing or contradictory) expansions of what justice or beneficence might mean in practice.

When considering the possible influence of theoretical bioethics on organization ethics, there is no reason we could not shift the focus of principlism from the individual level of the clinical setting and the physician-patient relationship, to the organizational level instead. If we do so, we find that the principles suggested by Beauchamp and Childress are useful in many of the same ways: they highlight generally agreed upon guidelines for action, and may provide a basis upon which agreement can be reached about issues in dispute.

Beneficence and nonmaleficence in clinical ethics practice are usually taken to imply that clinical decisions should be in the best interest of the person most affected, the patient. Thus they tend to reinforce the Hippocratic professional commitment to the individual patient. Beneficence and nonmaleficence can also apply to organizations, insofar as it is appropriate to maximize the well-being of the people whose lives are affected by the HCO, including all stakeholders, with particular attention to those for whose service the organization exists (in the case of the HCO, the actual and potential patients and patient groups). Justice seems as appropriate an ideal or operating principle for an organization as for an individual; that is, it can serve as a general and widely applicable evaluative norm, which we can apply not only to organizations in their relations to other organizations, but also on the other levels. Social expectations of distributive justice, for instance, remind us that it is important to continue to strive to arrange for equitable access to the social good of basic health care. (At the same time it is important to remember that this is a wider social obligation for which the HCO does not bear sole responsibility.) Autonomy, often interpreted as respect for persons, certainly represents a possible candidate for a "moral minimum" of the sort recommended by Walzer in our discussion of him in Chapter 2. Although it may be unclear what constitutes the appropriate positive expression of this ideal, we all recognize and could agree upon some breaches of it. An organization which does not provide appropriate medical care to the patients it serves, mistreats its employees, or exploits its contractual partners would be generally agreed to be manifesting lack of respect or disregard for the rights of the individuals and institutions to which it has responsibilities.

The criticisms leveled against principlism in clinical ethics—that it does not give definitive enough answers to practical questions, that it does not hierarchically order the principles that it invokes, that it is too theoretical or abstract and does not take proper cognizance of particularity, context, or relationships—are no less, and no more, applicable to its use by organizations. Although our practice-based, pluralistic approach does not encourage us to pursue it in this book, we can imagine the possibility of developing a principlistic version of organization ethics that might prove as vital, versatile, and adaptable to institutional ethical issues as the Beauchamp and Childress version of principlism has proved to be in bioethics.

Casuistry

Historically, casuistry grew out of an Aristotelian and medieval tradition, and several contemporary treatments of casuistry in bioethics link it specifically with Aristotle and his treatment of practical reason (Jonsen & Toulmin, 1998; Kuczewski, 1997; Miller, 1996). It fell out of favor as a method for moral reasoning with the growth in the early modern period of a more scientific turn of mind, and it is clear that its revival in recent ethical thought is not entirely independent from a growing skepticism about the value of a purely rationalistic approach to ethics. That ethical conclusions are at best probable, rather than certain, has become an acceptable and commonplace attitude rather than a reason for seeking a more rigorous method.

A casuistical strategy focuses on the practical solving of moral problems by a careful analysis of individual cases. A number of different approaches can be subsumed under this general heading, which at its least specific only implies reference to actual cases. There is a wide range of what counts as a case in the conventions of various disciplines, ranging from tightly crafted imaginative dilemmas in philosophy, to lengthy investigative explorations in business ethics; in bioethics the cases tend to be drawn from actual clinical or legal experience.

Casuistry approaches a problematic case by drawing analogies with other cases which resemble it in some relevant respects but are clearer in other respects, and thus can lend moral guidance. The elucidating case can be drawn from legal precedents, clinical experience, or even from artificially constructed paradigmatic examples. Moral principles may be used in casuistry, but they can have a more flexible status. Principles used by casuistry derive from actual practices refined by reflection and experience, and are always open to revision and further reinterpretation as new cases are considered (Jonsen & Toulmin, 1998). Typically they are treated as products of moral induction, rather than sources for deductive moral prescription, featuring in casuistry as concrete moral directives, maxims, or rules of thumb.*

---

*This qualified status of moral principles is often expressed by saying they express only prima facie, rather than absolute, moral norms. Cf. Beauchamp & Childress, 1994, p. 33.

Casuistry is preeminently a method for reaching decisions. There is a wide range of methodological recommendations for decision-making procedures in clinical ethics, many of which describe themselves as "casuistical," with various qualifications. Baruch Brody, Mark Siegler, and David Thomasma all have variations of an approach which promotes sound ethical decision making by concentrating attention on how a decision is made, rather than to what widely acknowledged moral principles it might represent. Part of the popularity of casuistry among clinical ethicists is no doubt due to the similarity of that method of reasoning to medical practice itself, which is case focused.

If casuistic approaches are useful for teaching and learning in other applied areas, the same will undoubtedly be true in organization ethics, since it is undeniably an area of applied ethics.

Virtue and character

Virtue and character ethics focus on the agent, rather than giving ethical primacy either to the consequences of actions or their characteristics. What makes an action good (virtuous) is not any particular characteristic of the action, but rather that it is the action of a particular kind of agent. One who is disposed by character or training to have appropriate motives, desires, and intentions is the basic model of the moral person. Professional ethics is a special application of virtue ethics. What most doctors still understand by medical ethics includes emphasis on personal traits like honesty, benevolence, trustworthiness, or fidelity (Drane, 1994, p. 28).

As well as good intentions, good judgment is a characteristic of the moral agent as defined by virtue ethics. The analysis of cases central to casuistry requires judgmental virtues such as vision, discrimination of morally salient characteristics, experience, and a range of skills often abbreviated, following Aristotle, as "practical reasoning."* The revival of casuistry and its increasing importance in clinical ethics is both cause and consequence of what one contemporary commentator calls "the revival of interest in ancient 'practical philosophy,' a turn to Aristotelian ethics on a number of fronts" (Kuczewski, 1997, p. 1) that sees a combination of virtuous character and seasoned practical reason as the most likely source of the kind of good moral judgment that is most useful in the clinical setting.

Early medical ethics considered good character necessary for excellent ethical practice, and that may be as true today as it ever was. But it also seemed to consider it sufficient. According to this ideal, good professional training in the hands of an ethical mentor should allow the ethical problems that arise in medical practice to be resolved by looking inward to one's character as shaped by the stan-

---

*Martha Nussbaum provides an interpretation of Aristotle's practical reason which is very useful for bioethics in a chapter of *Love's Knowledge* (Oxford: Oxford University Press, 1991).

dards and expectations of the profession itself. If that was true in the past, it certainly is not true today. The extent to which excellent ethical practice requires acknowledgment of the expectations of the society in which the professional practices, and the accommodation of professional standards to those expectations, is sometimes ignored.* The role of good character, of honesty, trustworthiness, benevolence, and fidelity, becomes that of the moral minimums discussed in Chapter 2—still necessary, but not sufficient for either success or happiness unless the environment in which we practice is such as to allow, and reward, only virtue. The profession of nursing is more realistic about the sufficiency of professional ethics. The history and the literature of nursing is rife with sensitive and often anguished discussions of the difficulty, and often the high cost, of maintaining professional virtues in environments hostile to them. We discuss these issues at greater length in Chapter 5.

What of virtues and organization ethics? High moral standards and ethically sensitive professionalism on the part of every individual occupying a role in a HCO would certainly contribute to organizational excellence, and the ethical climate of an organization composed exclusively of such individuals would have a good chance of having a decent ethical climate. But an important part of our motivation in attempting to formulate organization ethics is our conviction that because of the interrelation of the individual, the organizational, and the social levels of moral agency as described in Figure 2.1, individual virtue and character are not sufficient. Indeed, if the total responsibility for ethical behavior of organizations depends on the moral character of the individuals within the organizations, and no attention is given to the conditions under which they are expected to perform, we are more likely to produce martyrs and scapegoats than excellent organizations. We need to acknowledge, and to minimize as much as possible, organizational constraints upon moral action. We need to focus on the question of how to structure the HCO, and what strategies and procedures to build into them, in order to maximize the possibility of moral action of, and within, organizations. Our suggestion in Chapter 2 was that the internal ethical climate of an organization was an analogue on the organizational level of character in the individual. It is in this suggestion that the importance of virtue and character for organization ethics lies.

Ethics of care and clinical pragmatism

Feminism, nursing ethics, and most recently bioethics have developed versions of an ethics of care. Springing from early feminist roots, ethics of care in all its vari-

---

*We do not intend by the phrase 'accommodation' to suggest compromise in any morally problematic sense, but only to acknowledge that the application or interpretation of what any ethical principle means in a given situation is not always obvious. The Hippocratic prohibition of "using the knife," for instance, has been correctly assumed to be no longer relevant; this represents an accommodation to changing medical possibilities and an appropriate expansion of role.

eties focuses on relationships, context, and specificity of individuals and situations, and emphasizes the importance of perceptions and sentiment, as well as reason, in moral deliberation. Beauchamp and Childress have described ethics of care as relationship-based accounts, characterized by "an emphasis on traits valued in intimate personal relationships, such as sympathy, compassion, fidelity, discernment, and love. Caring in these accounts refers to care for, emotional commitment to, and willingness to act on behalf of persons with whom one has a significant relationship. Noticeably downplayed are Kantian universal rules, impartial utilitarian calculations, and individual rights" (Beauchamp & Childress, 1994, p. 85).

Many versions of ethics of care emphasize qualities that are also important to clinical ethics: concreteness, respect for complexity, particularity and ambiguity, and the centrality of the particular situation of the patient. In addition, good health care, both medical care and nursing care, are ethical enterprises, and, by describing them as *care* ethics, the importance of emotionally sensitive and responsive involvement with patients is underlined. Care ethics has been important to nursing ethics because insofar as nursing is professionally defined by the care of patients rather than specifically the medical treatment of patients, ethics of care validates the aspects of patient care closely aligned with nursing. It has been important to the broader bioethics enterprise by justifying its attention to the emotional aspects of clinical care. The ethics-of-care perspective has been criticized as claiming that only the affective or individualized aspects of clinical care are important, and writers from a variety of ethical traditions have suggested ways in which the insights and priorities of ethics of care can be accommodated within consequentialist (Kuhse, 1997) or deontological (Friedman, 1987) ethical approaches.

Pragmatism, or neopragmatism, a mainstream philosophical preoccupation for several decades, has recently attracted attention in clinical ethics as well, and like feminist ethics, it has been valued as much for what it opposes as for what it recommends. Clinical pragmatism assumes that the objective of clinical ethics is to resolve ethical problems that constitute an impediment to the plan of care for an individual patient. Its objective is not to work out the implications of any particular ethical theory for this situation, or even to isolate the particular principles that are most important, though in some cases doing so may resolve the problem. To that extent it is particularistic and pluralistic, as well as antitheoretical. It does resist compartmentalization of ethical considerations. Our assumption throughout this book that all actions and decisions, whether on the individual or organizational level, have ethical implications is very much in the spirit of pragmatism. Our insistence that what makes a decision or action ethically positive must include a reference to the particular situation and the context in which it occurs is given in the same spirit. These claims seem much more the expression of common sense than the imposition of any theory, even such an antitheory theory as pragmatism; but both pragmatism and neopragmatism make a big point of valorizing common sense, and claim to be a way to make common sense work.

Practically any theoretical approach to bioethics provides better direction for how to resolve ethical issues in clinical practice than does clinical pragmatism. This is the criticism most frequently leveled against pragmatism in all its forms, and it certainly applies as well to clinical pragmatism. If pragmatism does not give firm directives, it does justify and encourage both pluralism and flexibility. Pluralism of ethical approaches encourages the use of materials provided by theoretical bioethics from all perspectives as tools for resolution of ethical problems at the bedside; and if one tool does not work, the clinical ethicist keeps looking until he finds something that does work.* Flexibility is the refusal to be limited to one theory, one method, one approach, and is a corollary of pluralism.†

The approach to organizational ethics which we are recommending in this book is a pragmatic approach, with many of the weaknesses (as well as the strengths) of any other application of pragmatism. The objective of organization ethics as we understand it is to recognize ethical problems which arise in the course of organizational delivery of health care, and to try to develop mechanisms for addressing them. We do not have one answer to all questions, or even an expectation that all problems will have an answer. But we are convinced that today there are problems which need to be, and can be, addressed by adopting an integrated and integrating organizational perspective, and that we can find mechanisms which will further this project.

If theories are not central to a pragmatic approach, methods might be, on the understanding that any method (like any theory) is merely a suggestion about how to begin thinking about the problems confronted. In Appendices 2 and 3 we offer two alternative pragmatic approaches. One is the approach recommended by one of our authors to problems in business ethics, which may prove useful in organizational contexts as well. The other, the first twelve-step program for bioethicists, was developed for application on the social level, but can be applied on the organizational level as well.

As clinical ethics has developed, it has become basically a pragmatic endeavor focusing on mechanisms and activities rather than theoretical considerations. Much more consistent than the adherence to one or another theory, among clinical ethicists there is a pervasive skepticism toward *all* theory. Procedural recommendations for dispute resolution and decision making have been more readily welcomed in this area than any abstract theories. Because of what it does and who does it, clinical ethics is less concerned with the general issues of theory than with the

---

*This pragmatic "toolbox" approach to ethical theories was persuasively argued by M.C. Cooper in the context of the relation of justice and care in nursing ethics. See Reconceptualizing Nursing Ethics, in *Scholarly Inquiry for Nursing Practice*, 4(3), 1990. pp. 209–221.

†Judith Andre has suggested that Principlism was best understood in a similar way. Rather than a theory, or even a metatheory, the import of Beauchamp and Childress' approach was to provide a common language, similar to a trade pidgen, in which people with differing ethical presuppositions could nonetheless find enough common ground to seek agreement. (Andre, 1998)

specificity of cases. It focuses most explicitly upon the particularities of individual cases and the contextual factors including the important questions of who should be involved in the decision-making process and who is most affected by the decision being made.

SOCIAL CHANGE AND CRITICAL SOCIAL THEORY

Much has been written about the "birth of bioethics" as a social phenomenon. One popular view understands it as a widespread social response to what were perceived as abuses of medical practice, particularly the strong paternalism of physicians, in the middle decades of this century (Rothman, 1992; Jonsen, 1997). Factors frequently mentioned as both initiating and influencing the development of clinical ethics include a variety of social activism movements focused on particular "rights" of specific groups, and the rapid expansion of medical technology that created possibilities for medical treatment that had not existed earlier.

No matter the underlying reason, public concern and scrutiny of medical care has expanded to match the expanding impact of medicine on daily life. Health care and all that surrounds it have become a major social force in our culture. Healthcare professionals have always accepted moral responsibility for medical treatment; but increasingly the expectation has been that the responsibility will be exercised in public and explicit dialogue, rather than in the relatively protected privacy of the physician's office. Scientific and technological medicine, as one commentator has noted, "moved medical treatment procedures into the public forum" (Drane, 1994, xi). The healthcare provider is expected to say more; to say it in a less explicitly scientific language; and to say it in a dialogue in which recipients of care and their families are more explicitly involved than they were in earlier decades. Other social issues such as patient and family rights and values are important to clinical ethics, and clinical ethics specifically notes that professionals are not the only individuals with a moral stake in clinical decisions. It is committed to the social principle of shared decision making.

THE PRACTICE OF CLINICAL ETHICS IN THE HCO

Approaches to clinical ethics have undergone many changes during its development. We will consider some of the more important changes that have had an effect on clinical ethics today. Then, we will consider its role in contemporary patient care.

In response to a series of laws, regulations, and accreditation standards, HCOs have instituted, either voluntarily or under duress, a variety of committees and procedures designed to oversee various aspects of ethical medical practice within

HCOs. This history demonstrates a widening scope of ethical considerations in HCOs, but a scope that has been limited, until recently, to issues associated with the care of a particular patient or group of patients.

First came legislation addressing issues in human subject protection in medical research. In 1966 the Public Health Service mandated a local process of prior group review of any research project submitted for federal funding.* Since 1974 there has been a series of federal legislative initiatives that require internal institutional oversight and protection for research subjects.† The usual form of such oversight has been the formation of institutional review boards (IRBs), for review of proposed research on human subjects. The major focus of this "prior review" has been to assure informed consent of research subjects as well as the ethical conduct of research in other respects. Other specialized IRBs have been developed in certain institutions to review research using animal subjects. In teaching hospitals and research centers there may be an additional committee or board that addresses misconduct in research or complaints about improprieties of research such as plagiarism, falsification of data, or priority of discovery.‡

In addition to IRBs for considering ethical issues in human research, a number of HCOs created institutional ethics committees (IECs) for considering ethical issues associated with medical practice in specified areas, such as treatment of newborns or interruption of pregnancies. Various courts, state legislatures, and federal commissions recommended the establishment of these committees at various times in the 1970s and 1980s, but had little to say concerning their specific activities. Since 1991, JCAHO, the primary accrediting body for HCOs, has required that each HCO it accredits have "a mechanism in place for the consideration of ethical issues arising in the care of patients as well as education on ethical issues for caregivers and patients."§ Some committees have been established in response to this mandate; others expanded the function of already extant committees within the institution with previously articulated specific mandates, such as neonatal care or review of cases involving choices to forgo life sustaining treatment. Today between 80 and 90 percent of all U.S. hospitals have an IEC or alternate mechanism designated to attend to clinical ethics. Since not all hospitals are research centers, it is fair to assume that the clinical ethics committees or alter-

---

*Surgeon General, U.S. Public Health Service, Department of Health Education and Welfare, "Investigations involving subjects, including clinical research: Requirements for review to insure the rights and welfare of individuals." PPO # 29, Revised Policy, 1 July 1966.

†National Research Act, Pub. # 93–348, 1974, requires that all research involving human subjects receive prior group review by an institutional review board.

‡U.S. Department of Health and Human Services, Commission on Research Integrity: *Integrity and Misconduct in Research*, Washington, DC: U.S. Government Printing Office, 1995, #1996-746-425.

§Joint Commission on Accreditation of Healthcare Organizations, *Accreditation Manual for Hospitals*. Oakbrook Terrace, IL: JCAHO, 1992.

nate mechanisms, as recommended by JCAHO, are the major ethical resources available to the majority of healthcare organizations.*

An IEC in a HCO may have several functions: education in clinical ethics for the physicians and clinical staff who serve patients in the HCO (and secondarily for the community served by the HCO); assistance with development of policies and guidelines affecting the care of individual patients; and ethics case consultation to assist with ethical problems that arise in the care of these patients while in the HCO.

The educational function of ethics committees, while often including recommendations about community education in ethical issues of concern to HCOs, usually concentrates on internal education: workshops, presentations, and discussions for clinicians operating in particular clinical areas. Thus critical-care units may focus on end-of-life treatments, neonatal units on previable infants or developmental impairments, and obstetrical units on maternal-fetal conflicts. Information about new policies, recent court cases, or recent local cases that have created or called attention to ethical dilemmas may be discussed in in-services, unit or grand rounds, or public forums. Ethics committees in hospitals typically establish libraries or files on publications in the literature about experienced or anticipated patient care issues, and make the materials available to practitioners in the various clinical areas. Education is often correlated with other ethics committee functions, including policy development, and an ethics committee may act as a resource to the larger institution on ethical issues surrounding the care of most patients, such as confidentiality, competence determination, consent and refusal of treatment, and end-of-life care.

The impact of hospital policies on patient care is so obvious as to need little comment. Some HCO policies serve as a bridge between federal and state regulations and standards of practice within the institution. The JCAHO requires policy statements and guidelines for many issues associated with patient care,† and it is these policies that have been until now the main area of concern for ethics committees. Since traditionally, clinical ethics committees have been comprised primarily of clinicians, their review of policies allows for clinical as well as ethical input into policy creation. Expanding the range of policies with which that group

*American Hospital Association. *1992 Statistical Guide* (Chicago: AHA, data collected in 1989). These numbers mean that at that time of 2,071 hospitals with more than 200 beds, approximately 518 did not have a committee and of 4,649 with fewer than 200 beds, 3,487 did not have a committee. Clearly, outreach efforts are needed in smaller hospitals.

†Among the issues on which the JCAHO requires policy are informed consent; use of surrogate decision makers; research or clinical trial decisions; refusal of medically indicated treatment; advance directives; pain management; confidentiality of information and security of patient property; complaint resolution, organ procurement and donation, and access to medical records. For an excellent discussion of the functions of ethics committees in HCOs see John C. Fletcher and Edward M. Spencer, "Ethics Services in Healthcare Organizations," in Fletcher et al., *Introduction to Clinical Ethics* (2nd. ed.) Frederick, Md.: University Publishing Group, 1997, pp. 257–285.

is concerned can bring that advantage to a wider range of institutional concerns. Since IECs already exist in HCOs, many have begun to consider issues that have broader impact than an effect on a specific patient's care, and have thereby begun to consider organization ethics issues.

Ethics consultation is a service provided by an individual or group to help patients, families, surrogates, healthcare providers, or other involved parties address uncertainty or conflict regarding value-laden issues that emerge in health care.* Ethics consultation is addressed by one of several mechanisms: by the hospital ethics committee, by a subset of that committee designated as ethics consultants, or by an outside consultant. Frequently the role of the consultant(s) is not to decide ethical issues, but to explore and offer advice about ethically acceptable options, relevant legal cases, or social consensus. Lawyers may offer ethics consultation in some hospitals; and decisions about what is right are often tempered by consideration of what the courts and local jurisdictions consider legal.

Facilitating communication and dispute resolution are central concerns of ethics consultation. The time pressures of care in a busy hospital setting can lead to failures of communication, which can produce problems. If patients or family members do not adequately understand reasons for care decisions, or if different members of the care team fail to communicate adequately with each other, misunderstandings and differences of opinion can loom disproportionately large. Acknowledging that other clinicians, patients, and families may have valid moral positions that must also be recognized, clinical ethics nonetheless frequently implicitly addresses its claims to the physician decision maker.

Clinical ethics has as one of its objectives the creation, in the ethics committee, of a forum in which, whatever the professional inequalities, there is a presumption of moral equality of all those who have a moral stake in the outcome of a clinical decision. At the same time, the clinical reality has been that the physician decision maker has (or has had until recently) virtually complete control over conditions of patient care. If disagreements or misunderstandings are clarified with that decision maker, satisfactory outcomes will result. For that reason, clinical ethics textbooks often read as lightly camouflaged professional medical ethics, a set of directives to the physician about what is appropriate or inappropriate use of clinical power. It is in the literature of nursing ethics, not of clinical ethics, that issues of power in health care and the impact of organizational structures on ethical decision making are most often explicitly addressed.

For some clinical decisions in HCOs, there has been a shift of power from clinical professionals to administrators. As the typical model for healthcare de-

---

*Only one bioethicist, physician Howard Brody, explicitly addresses clinical power at any length, in his book *The Healer's Power*; and it is not the inequality of power between care providers that is his major focus. Inequities of power between physicians and other clinicians is a frequent subject in nursing ethics, and has been discussed as well by non-nurse observers of the profession. See for instance Reverby, *Ordered to Care*, and Milosh, *The Physician's Hand*.

livery changes from fee-for-service to some variety of managed care, physicians find themselves increasingly in the role of accommodating organizational strictures concerning such issues as the range of available drugs and treatments, billing practices, access to health care, financial incentives to reduce utilization, and restrictions on access to specialists and full disclosure to patients. Rather than acting as the ultimate and unquestioned decision maker, the physician is now only one voice in clinical decisions. This shift is not always reflected in the composition of ethics committees, a problem for which this book hopes to offer practical remedies.

CLINICAL ETHICS AND ORGANIZATION ETHICS

Problems in clinical ethics are important for organization ethics in several ways. First, as we have noted several times, most clinical ethics problems have organizational *implications*. In the course of resolving a typical clinical ethics case, structural problems often surface, whether staffing issues, problems with the approved formulary, or the absence of a policy that will provide guidance to clinicians. Excellent clinical ethics practice will note those problems and direct them to the appropriate organizational components. Second, clinical ethics problems often have an organizational *analogue*. Confidentiality, disclosure, truthtelling, informed consent, and conflicts of interest are as important in organizations as they are in clinical encounters, but the organizational responsibility to those values cannot be limited to or reduced to their clinical responsibility. Insofar as organizations also are ethical agents, and instrumentalities of the society for health care, they are subject to many of the ethical expectations that the society has of individual providers, and it behooves them to pay attention to those expectations as well. We will treat some of the organizational analogues to clinical ethics issues later (Conflicts of interest, and the important issue of conflicts of commitment, will be discussed at greater length in Chapter 8). Finally, although we will not defend this claim here, it could be argued that many clinical ethics problems have organizational *causes*—because policies have been implemented or changed without consideration of the clinical implications; because organizational priorities or values have shifted without adequate information, education, discussion or negotiation with all affected individuals; because of inadequate communication between various stakeholder groups in the institution. Some of these issues will be discussed in the chapter on instituting an organization ethics program in an HCO.

The practice of clinical ethics is an important organizational obligation, and an important part of the expectations of the society and of various stakeholders of the HCO; it must be protected by the organization. Clinical ethics shares with professional ethics a value that is constitutive of the HCO as an organization: the primary value of patient care. It is not, however, able to operate without considering the organizational implications of its attitudes and activities. The practice of clinical ethics must be part of organization ethics practice, but not identical to it, and it must be integrated into the organization's ethical climate and be able to act comfortably within this context. Obviously, organization ethics as we conceive of it will also be the function within the organization for the development and maintenance of the organization's consistent ethical climate, including the responsibility for the activities necessary to fulfil this important function.

Like clinical ethics, organization ethics is not just an application of theories from philosophical, business, or even biomedical ethics. Instead, it is a practice-focused set of procedures and mechanisms to address ethical problems that arise in organizations that deliver health care. Many of those problems are not questions about how to understand or apply clinical or professional ethical obligations, but arise when clinical, professional, or business ethical obligations conflict or produce conflicting recommendations.

As we suggested, there are two important issues inherent in the interface between clinical and organization ethics.

1. Clinical ethics cases typically have organizational implications (and sometimes organizational causes).
2. Some paradigmatic clinical ethical issues—confidentiality, disclosure, truth telling, conflicts of interest, informed consent—have organizational analogues.

We noted that many of the issues most central for clinical ethics are organizational issues as well. Patient privacy and confidentiality of medical information, for instance, are not just questions of identification of patient charts, but issues that need to be addressed on an organizational level. What safeguards does the hospital medical information system have against unauthorized access to patient information? What protection for patient anonymity does the system allow for those who have authorized access? What happens to information gathered for administrative, epidemiological, or research purposes? Are lists of end users of various pharmaceuticals made available to commercial enterprises that may then sell that information? Disclosure is an institutional, as well as a physician-patient issue. What rules or conventions does the hospital follow in discussing financial issues with patients? What rules govern institutional disclosure of policies, proprietary information, or practitioner statistics to patients? Other institutions? The community? What conflicts of interest or obligation do their roles in the institution create for healthcare professionals in various administrative positions? The importance for an accessible forum to discuss such issues is as important for organizational ethical issues as it is for patient-focused ethical issues.

Finally, some issues that are appropriate for organization ethics to address—financial policies, contracts, marketing, financial viability, personnel issues, public relations—are not ordinarily currently addressed by clinical ethics committees, and many cannot be appropriately addressed by the usual range of members of clinical ethics services in the institution. Many of the issues that are most important for clinical ethics as well as organization ethics are not addressed by *any* of the components of the organization explicitly; those include the hierarchical structure of HCOs, power relations within HCOs, and the ethical implications of organizational routines and structures. Thus there is a dramatic need for a broader conception of ethics in HCOs.

CONCLUSION

In order to address adequately the issues of patient care, clinical ethics can no longer be limited to the case-centered interpersonal or interprofessional issues that have constituted its major focus in the past, and many clinical ethicists are calling attention to this expanded agenda. The changing healthcare environment, with its blurring of lines of authority, alteration of traditional roles, and the increasing impact of organizational issues on patient care, requires a new approach to the overall ethical climate within the HCO: a larger, more global vision of the elements of organizational life that affects patient care, and an attention to the entire healthcare organization as the focus for the overall ethical climate. Clinical ethics is an important function of HCOs; but it must be reconceptualized as one of several crucial ethical perspectives; and fostered, integrated, and protected within this larger organizational enterprise.

4

Business Ethics and Organization Ethics

Business ethics, as an area of applied ethics, is the study of ethics and economics, the analysis of individual and company decision making, and the examination of codes, rules, and principles that govern business conduct. Business ethics also seeks to understand, describe, and evaluate business practices, institutions, and managerial actions in light of some concept of human good or human rights. Business is usually identified with certain utilitarian ends, e.g., profitability, economic sustainability, productivity, innovation, growth, and/or economic well-being, and ordinarily these are goals that also increase human satisfaction. A business that was unprofitable, engaged in risky choices that undermined its survivability, did not grow, or lost jobs for its employees would be judged as poorly managed and detrimental to human good.

We also appeal to other values in evaluating business decision making, actions, and outcomes: those of commonly accepted morality. A firm that consistently mistreats or does not respect its employees, that engages in unfair business practices, cheats its suppliers or customers, wantonly pollutes, or misrepresents its assets and liabilities is judged to be a bad company. Managers that perpetuate these practices, even if they are within the letter of current law, are judged to be morally bad managers. On the other hand, companies that do more than what is minimally required by law or morality, companies that promote human rights, institute equal opportunity in the workplace, develop environmentally sustainable and safe products and production or distribution processes, promote competition, and advertise honestly are judged to be excellent companies by business ethics standards. The best companies are those that flourish economically within a range of acceptable or even exemplary moral behavior; indeed, according to a recent study, those are the companies that are most likely to survive the longest in changing political, economic, and moral environments (Collins & Porras, 1994).

As normative applied ethics, business ethics evaluates business practice and decision making in light of standards and codes, it develops rules and codes appropriate to the context of commerce, and it offers a framework of moral reasoning to think through recommendations and solutions to ethical dilemmas in business. As evaluative, business ethics seeks to develop and use sets of normative rules of conducts, codes, standards, or principles that govern what one ought to do in particular business contexts, where the well-being, rights, or integrity of individuals or organizations are at stake.

Business ethics is also descriptive. It analyzes the moral development of managers and how they behave. It describes and compares companies, corporate cultures, the integration of ethics into managerial decision making, the role of codes and other authorities, and the effect of corporate sentencing guidelines and other government regulations on corporate activities. Descriptive business ethics also investigates causal relationships between individual moral beliefs or corporate statements of value and human behavior at work. In this chapter, as throughout this book, we will focus primarily on normative business ethics. But we do not wish to dismiss descriptive studies that play an important role in describing relationships between managers, professionals, organizations, governments, cultures, and even the environment, as well as describe how these relationships affect individual and corporate choices and actions. Indeed, it is usually difficult to cleanly separate out normative and descriptive content, because descriptive studies provide the information necessary for proper normative judgments.

There are many parallels between for-profit corporations that are not HCOs and HCOs. HCOs, whether they are nonprofit or for-profit concerns, are increasingly operating in a competitive business environment, and are subject to demands for economic sustainability (if not profitability), productivity, efficiency, innovation, customer satisfaction, growth and economic stability—demands that drive businesses. HCOs are ordinarily more complex than many businesses, however, in that the economic criteria which evaluate the success of many businesses, while also necessary for HCOs to meet, are never sufficient tests for the excellence of a HCO. Other criteria, both internal and external to the HCO itself, are equally relevant. A profitable, productive, growing HCO may still fail, morally, if the professionals it employs do not meet high standards of competence, if its actual level of healthcare service does not match the expectations created by its projected standards, if it does not serve the community population adequately, or if it redefines its obligations without community consensus.

Although HCOs are not identical to other non-healthcare-related businesses, the work done in business ethics on the nature of the corporation, on analyzing the nature of systems, on various kinds of evaluation and on management practices, constitutes a trove of knowledge that can be mined for the tasks of organization ethics. Business ethics provides us with various models for understanding decision processes in business. Several of those models are very useful for understanding the HCO: rational choice theory, integrated social contracts theory (ISCT), stakeholder theory, and other theories that link business ethics to more traditional models of theoretical ethics.

RATIONAL CHOICE THEORY

Some time ago, the Nobel prize–winning economist Milton Friedman declared: "There is one and only one social responsibility of business—to use its resources and engage in activities designed to increase its profits so long as it stays within the rules of the game, which is to say, engages in open and free competition without deception or fraud" (Friedman, 1970, p. 126). This often misquoted statement does not advocate that "anything goes" in commerce. Law and common morality should guide our action in the marketplace just as they guide our actions elsewhere. Nevertheless, given that qualification, which is an important one, Friedman places primary importance on profit maximization as the role of business. Thus managers' first duties and fiduciary duties are to owners or shareholders. Ordinarily these duties are to maximize return on investment, although in some companies the mission statement directs managers to other ends as well.

Friedman's conclusion is based on a neoclassical economic model of rational choice theory. Rational choice theory is based on the assumption that human beings act primarily from interests of the self, that is, in their own self-interests, broadly conceived. For example, Mother Theresa could be described as acting on her interests, which were to help poor, ill, aging Indians to have decent treatment and a dignified end to their lives. She could be called a rational utility maximizer since all her work was directed toward maximizing her interests. According to most proponents of this view, it is rational to maximize your interests (or at least irrational to harm yourself or otherwise lessen your opportunities or devalue your own interests, all things considered) (Gert, 1990). When one acts rationally (and no economist assumes that any of us does most of the time), one acts to maximize one's interests, or long-term interests, all things considered. Rational choice theory identifies value with individual rational utility maximization. What is valued by each rational maximizer are his or her preferences or considered preferences, and positive outcomes including positive economic outcomes can be achieved by satisfying the most considered preferences, all things considered (Hausman & McPherson, 1996; Sen, 1987).

Rational choice theory has often been misinterpreted as egoism. But this is erroneous. There is a trivial sense in which all my interests are self-interests; I am the subject of my interests, so they are interests *of* myself. But I am not always the object of my interests; that is, not all my interests are *in* myself. I have other directed, altruistic or benevolent interests, and can cherish disinterested values as well.* The organizational analogue of rational choice theory would be an organizational rational utility model: that organizations act, or should act, if they are rational, primarily in their own interests. The assumption by economists such as Friedman is that what is in the "interest" of a commercial enterprise is maximization of profit. If we understand business organizations on this model, what is ethical is the maximization of the interests of shareholders, since they are the owners of the enterprise. Any activities that do not work toward this end are unethical, since they violate the considered preferences of shareholders and question the fiduciary duties of managers. Notice that if managers are themselves rational, and thus interested in their own utility, corporations must provide the proper incentives to motivate managerial interests to align with those of the company and its shareholders. Despite this alleged introversive organizational focus on itself and its interests, it is further argued that in a climate of free enterprise, when the playing field is relatively level, competition between businesses may act to regulate economic interests, increasing well-being by producing competitively qualitative goods and services at low cost.

Rational choice theory has also been influential in changing the model of contemporary healthcare delivery. The promise of managed care has been that commercial competition will be a sufficient mechanism to improve the efficiency and reduce the cost of health care, without imperiling quality. Yet there are a number of difficulties with rational choice theory, even as it applies to the practice of commerce or business; and, as we will see later, even greater difficulties when applied without qualification to healthcare delivery. First, this point of view takes as its model the individual decision maker and applies it to the organization or corporation, neither of which is capable of being considered in isolation from a social context. Sometimes neoclassical economists speak of each of us as if each was an autonomous individual who is able to make choices and act in a social vacuum, without being affected by, or in disregard for, the community in which we live. But as we suggested in Chapter 2, one's cultural, social, and historical background, including socially assigned or adopted roles, relationships and intimate connections, and the expectations of others constitute a part of the definition of the individual. Similarly, on the level of the organization, both the roles

---

*This distinction is illuminatingly discussed by Adam Smith in the *Theory of Moral Sentiments*. Although the model of a constrained rational egoist is often attributed to Smith, it is simply untrue. Smith is not an egoist, nor does he place emphasis on the autonomous individual moral decision-maker; he acknowledges the intrinsically social nature of human beings. Smith, 1976, II.ii.3.1)

assigned to the organization by the society in which it operates and the values and expectations of the constituent members of the organization must be taken into account in explaining corporate action.

Second, a plurality of values, and the possibility of acting in a disinterested or altruistic and benevolent way is as possible for organizations as for individuals. A case in point was the reaction of Johnson and Johnson in 1982 to poisoning of Tylenol capsules. The CEO of Johnson and Johnson, James Burke, decided to discontinue the marketing of the capsules, despite the absence of correlation between the event and the Johnson and Johnson manufacturing process, and in the face of the risk of loss of its then dominant market share in pain medication. Citing Johnson and Johnson's credo, the first line of which states "We believe our first responsibility is to the doctors, nurses and patients, to mothers and all others who use our products and services," Burke withdrew the capsules from the shelves and they were never again manufactured or sold (Smith & Tedlow, 1989).

Third, values are not equivalent to preferences, even rationally considered preferences. We may prefer things we value; but that does not mean we value them only because we prefer them. There are agreed-upon social norms and standards for judging behavior that are distinguished from what we in fact prefer to do. Though the judgments in some cases may converge (and it is itself a morally desirable enterprise to bring them into convergence), we need to be able to distinguish in evaluative terms between outcomes based on recognized values and those based only on preferences.

The neoclassical assumption appears to assume that there is no ambiguity or internal conflict about preferences. Even if rational individuals are never subjected to conflicts of values or preferences (itself an unlikely assumption), the same assumption cannot be made of the organization as moral agents. Few organizations, even purely commercial ones, have only one goal or objective. Conflicts of value must be approached differently on the organizational level. While an individual can reasonably be imagined to be content with the result of an action which maximizes her preferences or satisfies her most dearly held moral values, even at the cost of thwarting other preferences or values (for she is the winner, as well as the loser, of benefits), collective decision making of the sort which is represented by organizational policy has the potential to distribute satisfaction unevenly among the individuals (or structural elements) who constitute the organization. Thus rational choice theory, applied to ethical decision making on the organizational level, rides roughshod over the moral agency of the constituent members of the organization.

Though rational choice theory fails as a normative framework for business and business ethics, there is one sense in which Friedman's version might be useful in thinking about HCOs. HCOs are, at least in theory, created for one purpose: to minister to the health of patients and patient populations. If their mission is patient or population health, then as rational agents they should act so as to maximize the treatment and well-being of their designated populations. Rewording Friedman,

> There is one and only one social responsibility of a HCO: to use its professional and economic resources and engage in activities designed to treat and improve the health of its patient populations so long as it stays within the rules of the game.

One of the rules of the game in the present economic climate might be the proviso that an HCO must be economically viable, that is, minimally, it must break even or create the ability to pay its debts. Even HCOs who depend on charitable contributions or state funds are under such economic constraints. Another rule would be the practice of following legal and regulatory mandates. This formulation puts in perspective and focus the unique feature of HCOs that distinguishes them from other types or organizations, including for-profit non-healthcare related corporations, while appealing to a Friedmanesque rationale and justification for its actions. Actions of an HCO that do not maximize patient or population treatment, would, on this account, be irrational and indeed, morally wrong, given the mission of the HCO. Efficiency, productivity, profitability, economic stability, needs and interests of healthcare professionals, interests of insurers, government, or the community are important goals only insofar as they contribute to the primary aim of the HCO. Having said this does not diminish the complexity of an HCO nor the difficulty in achieving its mission in the present political, social, and economic environment, at least in the United States.

INTEGRATED SOCIAL CONTRACTS THEORY

In recent work Thomas Donaldson and Thomas Dunfee put forth what they call integrated social contracts theory (ISCT). First proposed in the seventeenth century by Thomas Hobbes, social contract theory rests on the idea that, in theory at least, human beings consent to join together in societies and at least tacitly agree to laws and regulations governing their behavior so that they can live in harmony and achieve their own ends in relation to others. In contemporary parlance, "All rational humans aware of the bounded nature of their own rationality would consent to a hypothetical social contract, encompassing a 'macrosocial contract', that would preserve for individual economic communities significant moral free space in which to generate their own norms of economic conduct, through actual 'microsocial contracts'" (Donaldson & Dunfee, 1995, p. 89).

Donaldson's and Dunfee's contribution to social contract theory is to argue that there are basic "hypernorms" that govern all social relationships. What those are is subject to debate, but norms such as not causing gratuitous harm, honoring contracts, respecting or at least not denigrating basic rights, treating people and organizations fairly are candidates for hypernorms (Donaldson & Dunfee, 1995, pp. 95–96). Such hypernorms provide the moral baseline for organizational action and also govern organizational interrelationships. Within particular societies, and by analogy, within particular organizations, there is what Donaldson and Dunfee call "moral free space," dictated by the community in question. Although subject to compatibility with hypernorms, communities and organizations can spell out specific norms, acceptable customs, and agreements among themselves. Again, on the micro level these are tacit agreements since one seldom sits down, in a community or in an organization, to spell out or vote on these arrangements.

There are at least three useful concepts from ISCT that are worth mentioning: the idea of a hypothetical social contract (or the expectations that follow from that idea), the notion of tacit consent, and the notion of moral minimums, an idea we discussed in Chapter 2. In our society we have allowed HCOs to come into being and operate because we believe in health care and in expanding and improving health care for a variety of populations in our country. Therefore one could conclude that there is a tacit social contract between HCOs and society to carry out a mission to provide good-quality health care, and we find ourselves angry when a HCO fails in its mission or becomes distracted with concerns for expansion or profitability that seemingly override the basic mission. ISCT explains the source of our anger and concerns, and helps to justify those conclusions.

On a micro level, there appears to be a tacit contract or agreement between patients and the HCO. Patients expect to be treated and to receive adequate treatment. That expectation, which is not always a written-out agreement between the HCO and the patient, arises out of the nature and mission of the HCO. Sometimes, too, depending on the HCO, society expects it to handle populations of patients, and imagines there is at least a tacit agreement on that score. ISCT helps to explain how unwritten expectations arise and why they often have moral force, particularly when they are not reciprocated.

Third, while the notion of a hypernorm is confusing, following Michael Walzer and others, thinking of hypernorms as moral minimums is appealing, an idea we introduced in Chapter 2. Moral minimums are invaluable as justifications for making and evaluating moral judgments that cross organizational, cultural, or ethnic boundaries, and they make possible organizational and role evaluation.

What is less helpful is ISCT's idea of a moral free space, a space that could allow the production of untoward actions within or between less than perfect organizations. Moral free space, for example, allows for the domination of role morality in the organizational and cultural domains. While role morality has an important function in organizations, as we argued in Chapter 2, one must be able to evaluate roles and role obligations by more-general moral principles than those merely generated by role norms in an alleged moral free space. The connection between role morality and more-general moral evaluations of those domains remains indeterminate, and ISCT does not thoroughly work out that link. In discussing organization ethics for HCOs we will be much more explicit than ISCT about what is acceptable on the micro level in the alleged moral free space within a HCO. Indeed, stakeholder theory tries to bridge those gaps by eliminating the micro/macro distinction altogether.

STAKEHOLDER THEORY

What Friedman sometimes neglects to consider in his description of a manager's fiduciary responsibility to shareholders, is an organization's obligations to other stakeholders, in particular, in business, to employees, managers, customers or clients, and the community. One could not run a business without employees and could not stay in business very long without customers nor exist at all unless the community accepted commercial activity. These stakeholders, and there are others, are important not merely because one could not exist or achieve profits without them, but also because they are individuals or groups of individuals—human beings with rights and interests.

Another approach to business ethics that takes into account the rights and interests of the broad range of individuals and organizations who interact with and are affected by business decision making is stakeholder theory. Stakeholder theory is a promising business model for organization ethics because it acknowledges a plurality of values and moral agency on different levels. The complexity of an organization, and the difficulty, as well as the importance, of establishing an excellent ethical climate within an organization, can be better understood on the basis of this theory than rational choice theory or ISCT. By calling attention to the variety of roles that can be occupied by individuals, all of whom have a moral stake in the organization, stakeholder theory can help to provide a framework for understanding and explicating the possibility of conflicts of value, of loyalty, of commitment, and of interests.

Widely defined, stakeholders are "groups or individuals who benefit from or are harmed by, and whose rights are violated or respected by, corporate actions" (Freeman, 1999, p. 250). In a modern business corporation the primary or most important stakeholders commonly include employees, management, owners/shareholders, and customers, and usually, suppliers and the community as well. Focusing more narrowly, a stakeholder is any individual or group whose role relationship with an organization

1. "is vital to the survival, and success [or well-being] of the corporation" (ibid.), or
2. helps to define the organization, its mission, purpose, or its goals, and/or
3. is most affected by the organization and its activities.

In the first instance, stakeholder theory appears to be primarily descriptive; stakeholder relationships outline organizational role relationships within and outside the firm. Under the narrowly defined version, stakeholders appear to be those who are instrumental, one way or another, to the firm and its well-being (Donaldson & Preston, 1995). Prioritizing stakeholders helps to sort out and clarify organizational priorities so that not every person, group, or other organization affecting or affected by the organization in question is equally important as a stakeholder. Otherwise the theory is vacuous. To prioritize stakeholder claims one examines an organization's purpose and mission, ranking stakeholders in terms of who has legitimate or appropriate claims, and who is essential to that mission and to the survival and flourishing of the organization.

The instrumentality of the prioritization, however, deals only with part of what is important in stakeholder relationships. It does not take away from the intrinsic value of each stakeholder's interests, according to proponents of stakeholder theory, and, in fact, the intent of stakeholder theory is largely normative. "The descriptive accuracy of the theory presumes the truth of the core normative conception, insofar as it presumes that managers and others act [or should act] as if all stakeholders' interests have intrinsic value. In turn, recognition of these ultimate moral values and obligations gives stakeholder management its fundamental normative base (Donaldson & Preston, 1995, p. 74).

Challenging the position that a manager's primary responsibility is to maximize profits or that the primary purpose of a firm is to maximize the welfare of its stockholders, stakeholder theory argues that the goal of any firm and its management, is, or should be, the flourishing of the firm and all its primary stakeholders.

The very purpose of a firm [and thus its managers] is to serve as a vehicle for coordinating stakeholder interests. It is through the firm [and its managers] that each stakeholder group makes itself better off through voluntary exchange. The corporation serves at the pleasure of its stakeholders, and none may be used as a means to the ends of another without full rights of participation of that decision, . . . Management bears a fiduciary relationship to its stakeholders and to the corporation as an abstract entity. (Evan & Freeman, 1996, p. 104)

Let us assume for our purposes that all stakeholders in question are individuals or groups made up of individuals. If stakeholder interests have intrinsic value, then, according to R. Edward Freeman, the father of stakeholder theory, in every stakeholder relationship, the "stakes [that is, what is expected and due to each party] of each are reciprocal, [although not identical], since each can affect the other in terms of harms and benefits as well as rights and duties" (Freeman, 1999, p. 250). Therefore stakeholder accountability relationships are reciprocal relationships.

Obligations between stakeholders and stakeholder accountability notions are derived on two grounds. First and obviously, stakeholder relationships are relationships between persons or groups of persons. So one is reciprocally morally accountable to various stakeholders just because they are people, e.g., to treat individuals with respect, play fairly, avoid gratuitous harm, and so on. What is distinctive about stakeholder relationships, however, is that these relationships entail additional obligations because of the unique and specific organizationally defined and role-defined relationships between the firm and its stakeholders. For example, an organization has obligations to its employees because they are human beings *and* because they are employees of the organization (Phillips, forthcoming). Conversely, because of their organizationally defined roles, employees have role obligations to the organization that employs them and its other stakeholders *as well as* ordinary moral obligations to that organization and its other stakeholders.

In HCOs these obligations become more complex. For example, a HCO has obligations to its employee-professionals

1. because they are moral agents,
2. because they are employees, and
3. because they are professionals and hired *as professionals.*

Conversely, healthcare professionals have role obligations to the HCO that employs them and role obligations to patients, to their profession, and its associations. They may also have role obligations to the communities they serve and to healthcare payers, *and* they have ordinary moral obligations to all of these populations as well.*

Acknowledging a plurality of moral agents, their interests, and reciprocal moral relationships, stakeholder theory appears to be immune to some of the objections raised to the rational choice model. But how does one evaluate various stakeholder claims with each other and with the profitability criterion Friedman and other economists advocate? Even not-for-profit HCOs must survive, and in the increasingly competitive healthcare climate, economic survival even for the most successful HCOs has become a critical issue. How does one prioritize economic sustainability in HCOs against other claims, in particular, those defined by the mission to patient and population health?

In evaluating stakeholder claims Evan and Freeman, two of the initiators of stakeholder theory, initially took a Kantian approach, arguing that because stakeholder relationships are relationships between individuals or groups of individuals, any decision must be one that affords equal respect to persons and their rights, valued for their own sake. A decision or action that used people as means for other objectives would not meet this Kantian criterion. Similarly, even though respect

---

*An HCO has different obligations to a healthcare professional who is hired to clean rooms than it does to a healthcare professional who is hired as a professional. In the former case the obligations are to the person as a moral agent and as an employee, not as a professional.

for property, and thus profits, are important objectives for business, one must be careful not to prioritize property as equal to respect for persons, according to this line of reasoning. Such prioritization leads to judgments that value corporate material goals over persons, a valuation that would violate this kind of stakeholder approach. In addition to autonomy and respect for individuals, procedural fairness, informed consent, and respect for contractual agreements, are means tests for stakeholder relationships. And in a properly constructed stakeholder arrangement, stakeholders should have viable avenues for self-governance and recourse.

Some thinkers such as Robert Phillips develop a standard of fairness as the normative basis for stakeholder relationships. This principle, derived from Rawls's theory of justice, argues that "whenever persons or groups of persons voluntarily accept the benefits of a mutually beneficial scheme of co-operation requiring sacrifice or conurbation on the parts of the participants and there exists the possibility of free-riding, obligations of fairness are created among the participants in the co-operative scheme in proportion to the benefits accepted" (Phillips, 1997, p. 57, italics deleted).

These formal considerations of such a fairness standard should provide a set of externally derived minimum guidelines or moral minimums for evaluating stakeholder decisions: for judging some of them morally acceptable or morally problematic. Decisions that affect various stakeholders must meet these minimum standards of respect for individuals, fairness of procedures and outcomes, informed consent, and availability of recourse.

BUSINESS ETHICS AND ORGANIZATION ETHICS OF HCOS

In the past, business issues in the HCO have been relatively insulated from clinical issues for several reasons. First, as we discuss at greater length in Chapter 6, the hospital at earlier stages of its development operated on a combination of charitable and equitable premises, allowing for providing care to often be separated from financial support. Second, the physicians, who were primarily responsible for clinical care, constituted an independent power nexus within the hospital and were governed by their own professional codes of ethics. In exchange for a great deal of control over their conditions of practice, they took almost complete responsibility for patient care. Thus clinical and professional ethics could to some extent be compartmentalized from the business issues—a much easier feat when, as in much of the last few decades, virtually all care was reimbursed from some source or other. Third, HCOs were not categorized as or treated as businesses, although of course they were presumed to be governed by the same expectation for good management as any other organization.

Today this separation of powers and of issues is less possible, for reasons discussed at greater length in Chapter 7. Still, in healthcare organizations there is a temptation to separate business issues from clinical or professional issues. Ethical issues in the management of the HCO are often distinguished from those that face its clinical practice, and those, in turn, are distinguished from the challenges experienced by the professionals who carry out that practice. In the current climate, economic goals and exigencies seem often to override other considerations. In business, too, where the business is not health care, the process of integrating and applying ethical standards to management practices can appear to be difficult, because economic goals and exigencies often seem to override other considerations. But this is a misperception. Ethical issues are as much an integral part of economics and commerce as accounting, finance, marketing, and management. This is because business decisions are choices in which the decision makers could have done otherwise. Every such decision or action affects people or relationships between people in such a way that an alternative action or inaction would affect them differently; and every economic decision or set of decisions is embedded in a belief system that presupposes some basic values or their abrogation. Similarly, as we shall see in the contemporary HCO, financial, clinical, and professional issues are all so interrelated such that one cannot neatly separate, say, the cost of an MRI from a patient's need for it or from the professional expertise that determines the desirability of that protocol.

Of the theoretical models we have discussed in this chapter, stakeholder theory provides an understanding of organizations and organizational accountability that best integrates financial issues with other considerations. Stakeholder theory assumes that the organization and all its stakeholders form a shared moral community; and it appeals to moral minimums or principles of fairness when evaluating organizational decisions. But even this finely differentiated account, in its original formulation, may also prove inadequate when applied to healthcare organizations without attention to several problems. Figure 4.1 illustrates a typical stakeholder diagram, as it might apply to a HCO. Unfortunately that diagram does not capture the intricate and complex stakeholder accountability relationships in a typical HCO, nor does it adequately prioritize patients and populations as primary stakeholders.

Indeed, several characteristics of the HCO complicate our understanding of it as a business, and therefore are complicating factors in applying stakeholder theory to HCOs.

Mission

Few corporations define their mission solely in terms of profitability. Earlier we saw that Johnson and Johnson's first priority is to its customers. Motorola's mission is based on what it calls "Uncompromising Integrity," "emphasizing the *value* of integrity and respect for people" (Moorthy et al., 1998, p. 12). Levi Strauss is more forthright, combining a number of goals, including profitability, in their mission statement, which reads, in part: "The mission of Levi Strauss & Co. is to

Government   *Employees*

Whales   *Spotted Owls*   *Disadvantaged*

> **Any individual or group that can affect or is affected by an organization's decisions**

Businesses   *Customers*   *Managers*

Stockholders   *Peers*   *Labor Unions*

Senior Citizens   *Suppliers*   *Historic Landmarks*

FIGURE **4.1.** Stakeholders. Adapted with modifications from the Arthur Andersen Program in Business Ethics' Seven Step Model for Moral Reasoning. © 1991 Arthur Andersen & Co. C.I.E.

sustain responsible commercial success as a global marketing company of branded casual apparel. We must balance goals of superior profitability and return on investment, leadership market positions, and superior products and service. We will conduct our business ethically and demonstrate leadership in satisfying our responsibilities to our communities and to society" (Katz & Paine, 1994, p. 24). What we learn studying business organizations is that the best organizations integrate other missions with the aim of profitability; according to a study by Collins and Porras, the best (longest surviving, most responsible, and most profitable) business organizations are those that do not focus on profitability as their primary missions (Collins & Porras, 1994). Still, whatever the mission, *a* goal of any for-profit business firm is the economic flourishing of its shareholders, or of its primary stakeholders. When the mission of an organization combines several goals, questions of ordering and priority often arise.

While economic survival (if not profitability) are obviously necessary considerations for the modern HCO in the present economic climate in the United States, subtle differences between HCOs and other business organizations remain. Like non-healthcare-related for-profit corporations, HCOs are engaged in other value-creating activities, including professional excellence of its medical staff, long-term organizational viability, community access, and, most importantly, patient and public health. What is strange is not that a HCO is concerned with efficiency, profitability or at least, sustainability. But the trouble begins when a HCO realigns its mission or creates an organizational culture in which efficiency, productivity, and profitability become the first priorities.

The overriding mission and rationale for the existence of healthcare organizations by definition is, or should be, the provision of health services to individuals and populations. This constitutive goal stands in an uneasy relation to economic ends. In a for-profit business organization, producing and selling a product or service yields a fee that normally results in a profit to the organization and that profit ensures organization survival, new capital for research and expansion, and so on. In theory (although not in practice) the more that is produced and sold, the more profit the organization enjoys. But in the HCO there is no such tight relationship between the rationale of the organization's existence and the conditions for its economic survival. Indeed, in some instances a HCO is rewarded for providing fewer services, if it denies service to very ill or elderly people.

Patient priority

In any organization, how one prioritizes value-creating activities determines the nature of stakeholder relationships. Patients, the consumers of the healthcare services provided by HCOs, have a privileged status among the stakeholders. It is true that in many excellent companies profitability is only one of a number of goals such as integrity, customer satisfaction, employee well-being, and respect for community. Nevertheless, no for-profit entity can stay in business very long if it *loses* money. So while customers may be a set of important stakeholders, they are not the only primary stakeholder. This is not the case in HCOs.* Figure 4.2 illustrates HCO stakeholder relationships where the patient is the primary stakeholder.

Separation of customer/payer and consumer/patient

In HCOs, recipients of healthcare services are usually not the payers. The correlation between consumers and payers is very different in this organization than in the usual business, and there is a crucial ambiguity in the stakeholder role of "customer." Various forms of insurance, employer-sponsored health plans, or government agencies purchase health coverage for the individuals and patient groups who are the actual and potential patients for a given HCO. This three-way relationship complicates accountability between the parties affected in healthcare delivery. Unlike the typical customer, the patient may have no choice to go elsewhere or to change providers. Even in those cases where the recipient is also the payer, the consumer/patient is often ill and vulnerable. Unlike ordinary customers, patients are not always able to exercise their choices coherently. Worse, the complexity of the rapidly changing healthcare system is often not explained, or not clearly understood. The vulnerable patient has no prior knowledge of what to expect, and has little or reduced capacity to complain or to affect care delivery.

*For this reason, as mentioned before in Chapter 1, several influential commentators have suggested that all healthcare organizations should be nonprofit (Christensen, 1996).

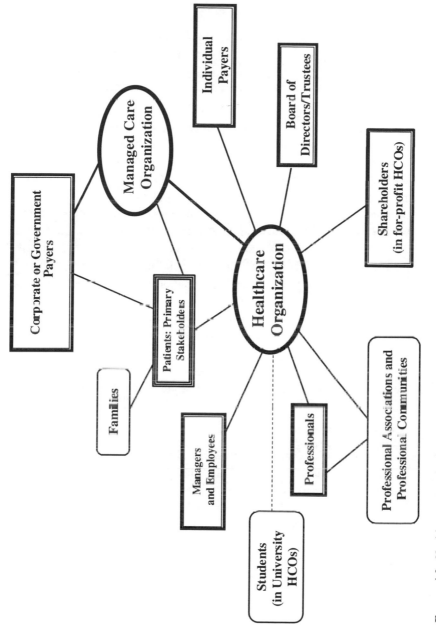

FIGURE 4.2. Healthcare organization stakeholder map.

Central role of professionals in HCOs

Healthcare professionals—physicians, nurses, members of other allied health professions—play key roles in the capacity of a HCO to deliver the services central to its definition and mission. It is the healthcare professional, not the manager, who is responsible for delivering care. One cannot gloss over, trade off, or subordinate professional commitments to patient health. Not only is this morally irresponsible for obvious reasons, it imperils the mission of any HCO, if an HCO is by definition a healthcare organization. Typically, healthcare professionals belong to, and are accredited by, independent professional associations. Many if not all professionals consider themselves primarily bound by the ethical prescriptions of their profession, preeminent among which are their duties to their patients. The necessity of professionals in HCOs complicates stakeholder relationships, particularly when the professional is also an employee of the HCO. Figure 4.3 illustrates stakeholder relationships from the point of view of the healthcare professional.

The complex accountability relationships between managers, professionals, and HCOs are not unlike managerial professional relationships in engineering firms since engineers, too, are specially trained professionals who belong to independent engineering associations. In both cases the presence of professionals complicates the organizational culture and in some instances may even challenge the professional to choose between her professional obligations and those to the organization. This is exacerbated in HCOs where there is an uncertain role for profitability or economic survival in face of the overriding commitment to health.

Contractual Arrangements

The contractual agreements an HCO enters into with managed care organizations and health maintenance organizations, with other HCOs, insurance companies, and affiliated professionals, and its Medicare and Medicaid arrangements, are increasingly important for the ability of the HCO to protect clinical and professional ethics. Today HCOs are expected to provide care to defined populations at reasonable rates and as efficiently as possible. HCOs have fiduciary obligations to the contractual payers for their services while at the same time they have primary role obligations to patients and populations. Moreover, if an HCO does not protect the integrity of its healthcare professionals it will fail in its mission to provide adequate health care and thus fail in its obligations both to patients and to payers.

Figure 4.4 illustrates the complex stakeholder interrelationships and accountability links in a typical HCO. What Figure 4.4 suggests is that while garden variety stakeholder theory (as illustrated in Fig. 4.1) does not capture the intricacies of HCO stakeholder relationships, a more complex version helps us to think through these intricacies and understand better relationships and how these rela-

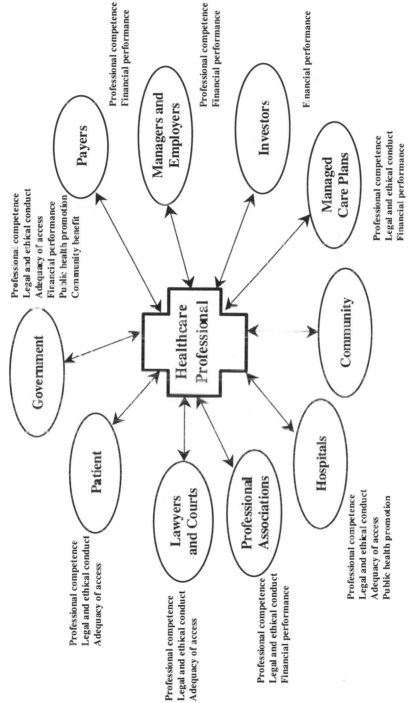

FIGURE 4.3. Accountability of the healthcare professional. This figure is a modified version of the figure used by E. J. Emanuel and L. L. Emanuel in their article "What Is Accountability in Health Care? *Annals of Internal Medicine,* 1996, 124:229–239.

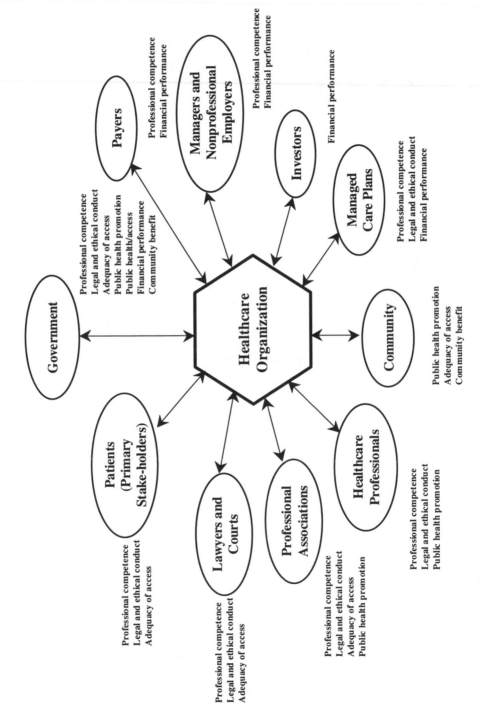

FIGURE **4.4.** Accountability of the healthcare organization.

tionships should be reciprocated. As we shall see in subsequent chapters, these various relationships often come into conflict with each other so that what in fact takes place belies our nice diagram. Still, setting out normative parameters for these relationships gives us a starting place to think about the ethics of HCOs.

CONCLUSION

Theories of business ethics, while developed in the first instance to analyze for-profit business organizations, are helpful in getting at ethical issues in HCOs as well. Milton Friedman's edict about social responsibility, when revised to specify the primary mission of HCOs, focuses attention on what HCOs are or should be about. Integrated social contracts theory brings attention to societal expectations for HCOs formed by implicit or tacit contracts between communities, patients, and these organizations. The notion of hypernorms or moral minimums gives credence and ground for external evaluation and self-evaluation concerning the culture, mission, and performance of HCOs, as well as the role obligations of their managers and professional staff. Stakeholder theory elaborates on the complex relationships between various stakeholders in HCOs, relationships that are some-times oversimplified in some delineations of HCOs. Stakeholder theory reminds us that stakeholder relationships are normatively reciprocal accountability rela-tionships prioritized by the organizational mission, roles and role obligations, organizational culture and climate, professional interests and obligations, moral minimums, and societal expectations.

In other respects, too, issues that business ethics raise are important to HCOs, particularly as they function as managed organizational providers trying to offer good health care as efficiently and productively as possible. Profitability is not always the only priority even in businesses unrelated to health and health care. There is no reason, then, to imagine that profitability should be the first order of business even in a for-profit HCO. The most exemplary for-profit corporations think about profitability as, at best, only part of their mission. Conversely, how-ever, separating business issues from those raised by clinical ethics or from the responsibilities of healthcare professionals may be detrimental to the HCO, to patients, and to the long-term professional commitment of healthcare specialists. This is because economic issues play a role in providing health care in every set-ting. Even in the "good old days" before managed care, healthcare professionals had to earn a living, and hospitals and clinics had to survive economically even on charity or governmental support. What is important for the ethics of HCOs is not to imagine that economic concerns are the only concerns or that profitability is the first priority, not that these concerns are irrelevant altogether.

Business ethics also reminds us that organizational accountability is as impor-tant as individual accountability. As it turns out, the HCO is at the same time a much more explicitly defined organization (in terms of its mission and clientele) and often a more complex organization (in terms of stakeholder accountability relationships, healthcare delivery, consumer/customer distinctions, who delivers services, and how these are reimbursed) than many other kinds of corporations. How one deals with the uniqueness and complexity of an HCO is the subject of the rest of this book.

5

Professional Ethics in Healthcare Organizations

We began this book with a number of assumptions, both theoretical and practical, that direct the scope and specific details of our work. These basic assumptions were outlined in Chapters 1 and 2. We acknowledge that there may be some controversy about each of them and wish to address one important area of controversy in this chapter: the relationship between organization ethics and the professional ideals of healthcare professionals. If organization ethics is to integrate the other ethical perspectives, it will have to encompass clinical ethics, business ethics, and in many ways the most important and most controversial area, professional ethics. In this chapter we will focus on medicine and nursing, but the conclusions are equally applicable to other healthcare professions as well.

In Chapter 1 we said that "HCOs are made up of healthcare professionals, managers, and other employees. They are responsible for patient and population health care, they have obligations to the healthcare insurers who ordinarily are not patients themselves, and they have duties to the communities in which they operate and serve. To be effective, organization ethics for HCOs must encompass a number of ethical perspectives, allowing and encouraging business, professional, and clinical imperatives to maintain their traditional stances when they can contribute positively to the ethical climate of the HCO." We assume then, that organization ethics should encourage attention and adherence to the traditional professional stance of the healthcare professional *when that stance furthers the ethical climate of the HCO.* The wisdom represented by professional codes and other aspects of traditional professional ethics should not be dismissed. These codes usually represent the very values upon which the ethical climate of an HCO should be based. But some aspects of traditional professional codes (particularly those relating to physicians) are not always helpful in addressing some common ethical dilemmas in today's healthcare world, where organizational and financial issues greatly affect decisions about the care of individual patients. "Ethical codes generally specify desirable consequences of physician behavior. However, it appears that such codes are of limited usefulness. It is more important to specify the organizational variables conducive to ethical behavior" (Crane, 1997, p. 195).

In some HCOs the longstanding professional principle that the welfare of the patient should always be primary is now being questioned since medical practices based on this principle have allegedly led to increasing costs. Situations in which possible benefit for one patient must be weighed against potential harm (or lack of benefit) to another have always occurred, yet each healthcare professional was left to make his or her own choices in these situations. Until recently decisions on budgeting and other financial issues, which sometimes cause conflicts of obligations, have been put aside by most healthcare professionals, who thus feel relieved of responsibility for any possible harms of those decisions on their patients. One often hears the excuse, "This is an administrative decision not a clinical one." As input from healthcare professionals on fiscal matters has entered more directly into these decisions, ethical conflicts have become more pressing. Yet professional organizations have had very little to offer their members struggling with these issues beyond the usual broad principles and guidelines from professional codes. Since decisions with financial implementions must be made and have significant ethical import, practical guidance is needed within the confines of the HCO where the healthcare professional is part of the clinical staff.

What do these changes in the roles of healthcare professionals imply? Will the familiar codes of ethics for healthcare professionals be replaced by an all-encompassing code of organization ethics that will define the ethical stance for the professionals associated with the HCO? How will healthcare professionals respond to such an endeavor? Would they be willing, as individuals or as a group, to accept the HCO as the source for professional guidelines and mandates, much as they have accepted professional associations as sources for these mandates in the past?

In this chapter we will explore these issues in more detail and present a model for modifying professional ethics so that it can function more affectively within the modern HCO and influence day-to-day decision making. We hope to point the way for a realistic reinvigoration of professional ethics that will be of value to individual healthcare professionals, to the healthcare professions in general, and to the individual HCO and its ethical climate as well.

WHAT IS A PROFESSIONAL?

There is no commonly agreed-upon definition of a profession or a professional. The term *professional* sometimes loosely refers to any person in a particular work-based group or to any person of authority. Indeed, we often use the word *profession* to refer to any group of individuals with particular skills who work from a shared knowledge base. Hughes (1963) comes closer to a working definition:
Professionalism may be defined ideally by four essential attributes:

1. A high degree of generalized and systematic knowledge.
2. An orientation to community interests rather than to individual self-interest.
3. A high degree of self-control of behavior through codes of ethics internalized in the process of work socialization and through voluntary associations organized and operated by the work specialists themselves.
4. A system of rewards (monetary and honorary) that is primarily a set of symbols of work achievement *rather than* ends in themselves. (Barber, 1988, p. 36)

Necessarily, a professional is a person who has had extensive and specialized training and has developed both specialized knowledge and particular practical skills. Part of the required training involves acquiring a skill or skills that will serve society or a particular segment of society in some way or another. The social utility of a profession is often embodied in its code of ethics or licensing process. Membership in many professions requires passing extensive examinations, and in most states professionals such as physicians and nurses must be licensed or certified in order to practice. Thus, being recognized as a professional is a privilege restricted by society and afforded only to those who are capable, trained, and licensed or approved in some other manner.

Almost all professions have their own organizations or associations. These organizations have codes that spell out the standards and expectations of a good practitioner, including the requirement of education and service to the community or a segment of the community. Development and maintenance of standards for ethical behavior are important aspects of the work of professional organizations. A few professional organizations, such as the American Institute of Certified Public Accountants (AICPA), serve in the capacity of examiners and grantors of licenses as well. To call oneself a "certified public accountant" (CPA), one must pass a series of AICPA-administered examinations and be certified by that organization. In this case, the professional organization defines what a CPA is, not only in terms of the personal and professional qualities that the CPA should possess, but also in terms of a very specific, state-sanctioned licensing process.

Professional associations are usually voluntary, independent organizations. At times, however, they have been used by entities outside the profession to define appropriateness for specific practice, which essentially makes belonging to the organization mandatory. From the 1930s to the 1970s, most hospital privileges for physicians in the United States were tied to membership in the local medical society, and many medical societies required membership in the American Medical Association (AMA).

The definition of a professional as applied to physicians, nurses, and other healthcare professionals obviously includes the factors we have been discussing, but there are important additional considerations. "In the classic sense being a professional implies a publicly declared vow of dedication or devotion to a way of life. It implies a special knowledge not available to the average person; it is an unequal relationship. But with that special knowledge comes a special responsibility. It is thus a fiduciary relationship in that the possessor of knowledge has a responsibility of altruism, and the recipient of the special knowledge may thus trust the professional. In other words a professional is a trustworthy trustee" (Orr, 1992).

The following characteristics have been included in one definition of a healthcare professional (Spencer, 1997b):

1. Arduous and very advanced training.
2. Well defined and circumscribed role.
3. Continuing education throughout one's career.
4. Control over admission to the profession by the profession (this has less relevance today than in the past but is still important).
5. Responsibility to specified individuals (patients) and either a defined or ill-defined obligation to a larger group (public in public health, community in other aspects of professional practice).
6. Devotion to humanistic ideals.
7. A well-defined group of necessary virtues and moral rules that define the ethical parameters of the profession.

Notice the emphasis on control, responsibility, and virtue, characteristics that were not a major emphasis in the previous definitions. Notice, too, how this definition intertwines special knowledge with special obligations. For many this is the essence of what it means to be a healthcare professional, particularly a doctor or nurse. In what follows we will argue that an organization ethics program in the HCO can support and enhance these essential qualities, while at the same time allowing the physician and nurse and the HCO to come to realistic terms with the decisions necessary for the organization to function effectively.

CONFLICTS OF INTEREST AND CONFLICTS OF COMMITMENT

A complex, difficult feature of professionalism is the level of autonomy of the practitioner in particular situations. Professionals are expected to exercise their expert judgment in their practice, and those outside the profession respect, if not agree with, that judgment. Professionals are expected to abide by their professional code of ethics, and indeed, this code is expected to override other considerations if a conflict should arise. Yet most professionals today are also employees or partners in a practice. As a result, organizational or partnership interests sometimes conflict with professional judgment or the demands of a professional code. In some organizations there is a perception that managerial or institutional priorities are assumed to take precedence over those of expert professional judgment, placing the professional in the difficult position of being asked to act in ways that violate or at least challenge her professional role as defined by the professional code (Bayles, 1981). These sorts of conflicts are ordinarily labeled conflicts of interest.

The Association of American Medical Colleges (1993) defines a conflict of interest as "any conflict between personal interests where acting with disregard to that conflict by placing one's personal or financial interests ahead of professional interests compromises or detrimentally influences professional judgment in conducting or reporting research." A conflict of interest refers to situations where one's profession, professional judgment, or professional code is in conflict with other demands or influences that, if acted upon, would compromise professional judgment. An organizational demand that questions one's professional judgment or conflicts with a professional code creates one such type of conflict. Conflicts of interest occur in every part of life as various roles conflict with others, where professional integrity is at question, when there are professional biases concerning judgment, or where demand for financial rewards, cost-cutting, or greater efficiency challenge one's professional decision making. Having a conflict of interest itself, however, is not unethical. It is only when one acts on that conflict in ways that break acceptable rules for sound medical decisions, that jeopardize professional judgment, or that cause harm that the conflict raises ethical issues (Werhane & Doering, 1995). Conflicts of interest cannot always be avoided. Still, in facing a conflict of interest one can appeal to certain guidelines to evaluate and mitigate the situation.

1. One should recognize and acknowledge the existence of these conflicts.
2. One should, whenever possible, disclose the existence of these conflicts to all parties.
3. Third, one should ask a series of questions:
   a. How would an impartial professional evaluate and act in this kind of situation?
   b. Would acting on the conflict of interest compromise one's professional judgment?
   c. What kinds of precedents would acting on this conflict set? Would you expect other professionals to act similarly? Can this be defended in a public forum?
   d. Who is harmed or benefited from acting on the conflict of interest?
   e. Can such actions pass the moral minimums test we suggested in Chapter 2?
   f. What kind of institutional structure, accountability procedure, or other constraint might have contributed to the existence of this conflict? Can those factors be mitigated in the future?
4. Finally, in unavoidable conflict-of-interest situations one may have to withdraw from the situation. If one cannot resolve clashes with an employer over the compromise of professional standards that seriously harm patients, a professional might have to leave that organization, and even, in some cases, blow the whistle publicly on that HCO.

Conflicts of interest are usually distinguished from conflicts of commitment, although they overlap. "Conflicts of commitment are those sets of role expectations where competing obligations prevent honoring both commitments or honoring them both adequately" (Werhane & Doering, 1995, p. 61). Professionals with limited time and resources and a variety of professional demands often face conflicting professional demands that are impossible to honor simultaneously. Professionals cannot always serve the needs of every patient or serve them well; they constantly face conflicts between research and clinical demands or service to the profession. Conflicts of commitment also arise as role conflicts. In a complex society each of us has a number of roles, and inevitably they clash. One simply cannot honor all one's commitments as a parent, spouse, citizen, professional, manager, and employee satisfactorily all the time. Unlike conflicts of interest, one can neither avoid the existence of conflicts of commitment nor avoid acting on those conflicts unless one simply abrogates all one's duties altogether. As a healthcare professional and as an employee, conflicting demands that hurt patient care are forms of conflicts of commitment between role demands as an employee and as a professional. Ordinarily, however, these demands are more complex. A professional may be faced with limited resources and the decision as how to best allocate them over a defined patient population. In such cases the professional commitment to serve each individual patient is constrained by the need to serve other patients, thus creating a conflict of commitment. A healthcare professional with a large caseload has always faced conflicts of commitment in deciding which patients have the greater needs of her time and services.

How should one deal with conflicts of commitment?

1. Again, as with conflicts of interest, disclosure and publicity are essential elements. A patient (or a patient population) who is cognizant of the demands of a healthcare professional where the limits of what will be provided are spelled out, is much more understanding of her treatment, for instance, than one who is unaware of this.
2. One often has to perform "triage" on commitments: prioritizing them in terms of who is least harmed or most benefited, which demands are necessary for professional excellence, which least violate one's other role commitments, and which can be put aside.
3. There may be organizational structures or accountability procedures that create conflicts of commitment. These must be addressed and changed.

Organizations, too, face conflicts of interest and conflicts of commitment. These are created both by conflicts faced by professionals and others working in or for the organization and by the organizational structure, mission, or climate. For example, professional conflicts of interest and commitment continue on an organizational level in HCOs and are sometimes exacerbated if there is pressure to increase numbers of patient contact, thus creating both professional and organizational conflicts of interest and conflicts of commitment. If the mission of an HCO is to provide health care for a defined population, then limited resources place it in an almost perpetual conflict of commitment situation. An HCO that alleges its mission is to serve patients, yet prioritizes profitability, places itself and its managers in a conflict of commitment as well as a conflict of interest. Such an organizational culture usually creates conflicts of commitment for professionals in the organization as well.

This is not to imply that organizations always make the wrong choices, merely to point out the pervasiveness of conflicts of interest and commitment.

A case that illustrates conflicts of commitment, role conflicts, and organizational conflicts is the 1996 *Challenger* space shuttle explosion. Engineering codes contain the provision that the engineer's first priority is the safety of his product. The engineers at Morton Thiokol, who were responsible for the design and ultimate use of the O-rings on the Saturn rocket scheduled to send the *Challenger* into orbit on January 28, 1986, refused to sign off on the launch of the *Challenger* on the night before the launch. Low temperatures were predicted on the launch pad the next day, and they had not tested the viability of the shuttle O-rings, the rubberized seals in the connecting joint between two segments of the rocket booster, at temperatures below 50 degrees Fahrenheit. Thus, the engineers reasoned, they could not be sure whether the O-rings would perform satisfactorily. There was intense internal and external pressure on these engineers to change their recommendations, but they refused. The decision to launch despite the low temperatures was made at a higher management level by men who had been trained as engineers. Their decision was based on the premise that since the O-rings had not been proven to fail, there was no evidence they would not succeed. The subsequent explosion of the *Challenger* was due to leakage of fuel from the cold, and consequently brittle, O-rings.

PROFESSIONS, HEALTHCARE EXECUTIVES, AND ROLE MORALITY

As we suggested earlier, conflicts of interest and conflicts of commitment often appear as role conflicts. According to Alan Goldman, the distinguishing feature of professionals is that their roles are what he calls "strongly differentiated." Goldman contends that professional codes are moral demands to which a professional subscribes when he chooses to become a professional. As moral demands they take precedence in situations involving professional judgment even when other moral demands are at stake. When faced with conflicts of interest, a physician, lawyer, or an engineer is expected to uphold the code of his profession, even when the contemplated action might be questionable by other moral criteria. For example, a priest is expected to uphold the confidentiality of the confessor, and in some cases the lawyer of the client, even when that person has committed a horrendous criminal act. An engineer is expected to prioritize safety even when it conflicts with other organizational goals and activities. A healthcare professional is expected to put the well-being of the patient as the first priority even if doing so is counterproductive to the goals of the HCO (Goldman, 1980). For managers who are also healthcare professionals, the challenge is acute, because these people are always faced with *competing* professional and managerial demands that challenge their interests and commitments.

Following Goldman, we would argue that physicians and nurses are professionals in this closely defined sense. Goldman would argue that healthcare managers and administrators who are not also healthcare professionals are not. Managers are not professionals under this definition because:

1. Their training is not narrowly defined nor required for their position
2. There are no specialized examinations or licensing or certification procedures in order to become a manager
3. There is no independent body such as an association or organization that regulates the profession or its members;

4. There is not an agreed on code of ethics developed for and applying uniquely to managers
5. There is no explicit connection between managerial expertise and social responsibility or service to the community.

In Goldman's terminology, managers have weakly differentiated roles, that is, they are not faced with conflicting *moral* demands of a profession that affect their judgments as managers. Ordinarily, managers are expected to be loyal to, and maximize the expectations of, the organization they manage and the position they occupy in that organization. They are also expected to behave in at least a minimally morally acceptable manner and not be socially irresponsible. But ordinarily even these criteria are de facto expectations and not spelled out or reinforced by any independent association or licensing body. The only distinguishing recognizable characteristic of managers is that they are given the position of "manager"; they are expected to direct, in some capacity or another, and as managers, rather than employees, they are responsible for the well-being of the organization. While managers face possible conflicts of interest and conflicts of commitment, ordinarily the kinds of conflicts do not include conflicts related to professional obligations and do not include conflicts with their independent profession or professional association (Werhane & Doering, 1995).

One will notice that in the foregoing paragraph, we repeatedly used the term "ordinarily" in discussing the nonprofessional status of most managers. This discussion must be qualified when referring to *healthcare* managers. While it is true that ordinarily managers do not fit the criteria of professionalism, at least as the term is used technically, in healthcare organizations some healthcare executives have formed the American College of Healthcare Executives (ACHE). Membership in this association is voluntary, as it is in most professional associations, and it is not evident that membership is important to, or thought to be necessary for, all healthcare managers. Moreover, membership does not specify a requirement of any prior special education or training, and healthcare executives are not licensed by any independent government body.

What is interesting about the association, however, is that sections of its code of ethics read very much like the code of a traditional healthcare professional. The code (American College of Healthcare Executives, 1998) states: "The fundamental objectives of the healthcare management profession are to enhance overall quality of life, dignity, and well being of every individual needing healthcare services; and to create a more equitable, accessible, effective, and efficient healthcare system." Further, there is a virtue component in the code: "Healthcare executives have an obligation to act in ways that will merit the trust, confidence and respect of healthcare professionals and the general public. Therefore, healthcare executives should lead lives that embody an exemplary system of values and ethics," (p. 2).

Although the ACHE code does not prioritize stakeholders, according to the code, the healthcare executives' responsibilities are "to the profession of healthcare management . . . to patients or others served, to the organization and to employees" (American College of Healthcare Executives, 1998, pp. 2–3). These appear to be the primary stakeholders, according to this code. In addition, the code specifies that healthcare executives have responsibilities to the community and to society. There is no attempt to argue that the healthcare organization has priority as a stakeholder. The code discusses conflicts of interest between the healthcare executive as professional and personal financial interests, but it does not deal with conflicts of commitment. Still, the existence of ACHE and its clear mission and code indicate a possible trend in the professionalization of healthcare managers.

Most interesting is the education component of the ACHE. Although membership does not require prior specialized knowledge, there are three levels of membership, associate, diplomate (CHE), and fellow (FACHE). Each has minimum requirements for entry, and the latter two have stiff credentialing processes. To be an associate one should have a master's degree and one year of healthcare management experience, or a bachelor's degree and three years' experience. Both the CHE and FACHE require continuing education as well as advanced experience.

Much of the recent attention to organization ethics in HCOs may be related to what appears to be a lack of professionalization of HCO managers. The ACHE code and credentialing processes are first steps in mitigating some negative perceptions and outcomes. Organization ethics may be considered a further and more conserted attempt to introduce professional moral obligations to the organization as a whole, by forming and supporting a positive ethical climate within which the manager works. The ethics guidelines promulgated for the whole organization may be seen as a constraint on the work of the manager, just as professional guidelines in the form of professional codes are constraints on the actions of the healthcare professionals in the HCO. Organizational ethics guidelines should also help in dealing with conflicts of interest and conflicts of commitment by providing forums for sorting out these issues publicly, and helping in their resolution.

HISTORY OF MEDICINE AS A PROFESSION

To understand the importance of professional ethical mandates on the activities of healthcare professionals directly affected by these mandates, it is helpful to consider the history of the development of the healthcare professions, particularly medicine. The history of medicine as an ethical profession began with the Hippocratic school in Greece in the fifth century B.C. The Hippocratic oath is still considered by many to be the best single statement of the professional obligations of a physician even today. The set of mandates contained in it form a general statement of ideals and obligations focused on protecting the patient by appealing to the finer instincts of the physician. The oath includes a strong confidentiality clause, statements advocating honor for instructors in imparting specialized knowledge only to those who agree to adhere to the oath, clauses pertaining to benefiting the sick and keeping patients from harm and injustice, as well as admonitions against euthanasia and abortion (See Appendix 4 for codes of ethics from different professional organizations).

Admonitions against "using the knife" (in the original oath), and certain self-serving practices to limit admission to the profession have slowly fallen by the wayside. But, in spite of these and other minor modifications, the Hippocratic oath has remained the expression of ideal conduct of a physician and has served as the basis for codes of other healthcare professionals. The strong emphasis on beneficence toward the patient and on the acquisition and maintenance of competence are as important today as they were in the time of the Hippocratic school. Very recently, the longstanding prohibition on performing abortions and assisting in dying have been questioned. Those who oppose these practices use the tradition of Hippocratic medicine as one of the arguments against these changes.

Following the early Greeks, the professional ethics of medicine were linked to traditional values associated with Christian, Jewish, and Islamic religions. These influences encouraged the development of compassion and other humane virtues in addition to the competence and beneficence emphasized by the early Greek physicians. In this way, professional medical values were strongly influenced by religious values; medicine, like the priesthood, became a profession to which one could also be "called." With this emphasis it became common for the medical profession to be seen as a conduit for God's power in healing the sick.

In 1803, Percival published his *Code of Medical Ethics* which he called "a scheme of professional conduct relative to hospitals and other charities." Percival's guidelines were based on the Hippocratic tradition, to which he added a number of more mundane issues, emphasizing professional etiquette and specific admonitions. For example, Percival believed that physicians should "keep heads clear and hands steady—by observing constant temperance" (Leake, 1927).

The primary source of contemporary codes for healthcare professionals probably dates to the 1847 organizational meeting of the American Medical Association. There the AMA specifically addressed two issues of importance: minimum requirements for medical education, and the establishment of a code of ethics for American physicians. A few organized statewide medical societies of the time had written codes of conduct, but these were not focused on the physician as a professional with specific obligations to the patient. The "Principles of Medical Ethics" developed by the AMA at that time were loosely based on Percival's treatise and on the Hippocratic tradition. It was to some extent an exclusionary document which set specific educational, practice, and ethical guidelines for the practice of medicine (AMA, 1996). We have included the AMA's principles in Appendix 4, xi, but it has served as a model for other healthcare professional codes.

The AMA's initial "Principles" were unchanged until recently. In 1957 the format of the principles was changed to ten short sections, preceded by a preamble. In 1977, the AMA principles were again revised "to clarify and update the language, to eliminate reference to gender, and to seek a proper and reasonable balance between professional standards and contemporary legal standards in our changing society." In this manner the AMA began to respond directly to modern-day social forces that greatly affected the practice of medicine.

SOME BASIC ISSUES FOR PHYSICIANS AND OTHER HEALTHCARE PROFESSIONALS

Since the early 1990s the AMA has advanced a "Code of Medical Ethics" consisting of four related parts:

1. "Principles of Medical Ethics," which is the fundamental statement of the core principles of the code
2. "Fundamental Elements of the Patient-Physician Relationship," which for the first time spells out mandates for the physician in terms of the rights of patients rather than the obligations of the physician
3. "Current Opinions," which reflect the application of the Principles to well over 100 specific ethical issues in medicine
4. "Reports" on issues of importance and interest prior to or concurrent with the issuance of an "Opinion." (AMA, 1996, viii)

Most physicians believe that the ethical basis for medical practice is the traditional "calling" concept, with its connotation of a higher power and nonnegotiable principles, or, minimally, very slowly changing fundamental precepts that include the idea of perfecting oneself through one's work. If this is the basis for the ethics of medicine, an obvious question then comes to mind: Can the basis for ethical practice change over time as a result of changes in culture and the social milieu? At present, there is little overt argument on this point; most healthcare professionals accept the fact that social changes affect medical practice and to some extent the ethical basis for this practice. But the question remains, how much change is acceptable before one is no longer talking about a healthcare *professional*?

Many would argue that the concept of a healthcare professional, rather than grounded on a strong, unchanging tradition believed by many to be based on a relationship with a higher power, has developed as a contract with society. They contend that this social contract allows, or even requires, certain special privileges for the professional in return for a specific set of obligations and goals focused on the care of specific patients. Is the social contract the real source of authority for physicians and nurses and other healthcare professionals, or is the traditional view the appropriate ethical basis for medical practice? Embedded in this question is an important practical issue: To whom does a healthcare professional owe ultimate allegiance—to society, based on the contract, or to humanity as represented by her individual patients, based on her calling and the traditional principles? How one approaches this issue in the healthcare world today can have significant ramifications on professional guidelines and codes, on how legislative bodies and courts respond to healthcare issues and conflicts, and on where the final source for accountability for healthcare decisions will be located. Polls reveal that most patients believe it is necessary to re-enforce the traditional ideals so that the core values of the profession are maintained in a relatively unchanging manner. Even so, the social contract can be considered to outline some of the parameters of the calling in that it may define certain relationships to other aspects of society in today's world and thus foster a clearer understanding of the role of the physician. So, both the traditional concept of a calling and the idea of a social contract may be at work here. The calling provides the primary authority for the physician while the social contract defines relationships to other rapidly changing aspects of the society.

The seven principles now advanced by the AMA include calls for competency, honesty, respect for law, respect for the rights of patients and others, continuing study and cooperation with others who have specialized knowledge, freedom to choose one's patients, and recognition of a responsibility to the community. Nowhere in these AMA principles is there a specific statement concerning putting the needs of the individual patient above all other considerations, which had been the traditional stance of organized medicine until the early 1980s when the principles were last revised (AMA, 1996, xiv).

The American College of Physicians, in attempting to speak for the ethical basis for the practice of internal medicine as well as for the rest of the profession, has said in its Ethics Manual (American College of Physicians, 1998), "Medicine, law, and social values are not static. Reexamining the ethical tenets of medical practice and their application in new circumstances is a necessary exercise" (p. 1). In this manual, the ACP attempts to shed light on many ethical tensions faced by internists and their patients and on how existing principles extend to emerging concerns. Their manual is meant to serve as a reminder of the shared obligations and duties of the medical profession. The ACP goes on to say, "Some aspects of medicine are fundamental and timeless. Medical practice however does not stand still. Clinicians must be prepared to deal with changes and reaffirm what is fundamental" (ibid.). Major principles advanced by the ACP are:

1. "The patient-physician relationship entails special obligations for the physician to serve the patient's interest because of the specialized knowledge

that physicians hold and because of the imbalance of power between physicians and patients" (ibid.).

2. "The physician's primary commitment must always be to the patient's welfare and best interests, whether the physician is preventing or treating illness or helping patients to cope with illness, disability, and death. The physician must support the dignity of all persons and respect their uniqueness. The interests of the patient should be promoted regardless of financial arrangements, the health-care setting, or patient characteristics, such as decision making capacity or social status" (ibid,).

3. "The patient-physician relationship and the principles that govern it should be central to the delivery of care. These principles include beneficence, honesty, confidentiality, privacy, and advocacy when patients' interests may be endangered by arbitrary, unjust, or inadequately individualized institutional problems" (p. 26).

4. "Physicians must promote their patient's welfare in an increasingly complex healthcare system" (ibid.).

5. "Physicians should also contribute to the responsible stewardship of healthcare resources" (p. 27).

6. "The physician's duty further requires that the physician serve as the patient's agent in the healthcare arena as a whole" (ibid.).

The ACP strongly supports the primacy of the patient-physician relationship and the physician's primary obligation to her patient. It also recognizes the important necessary contribution of physicians to the proper operation of the healthcare system. To date, neither the AMA nor the ACP has developed a mechanism to address the potential conflicts of these two positions beyond the ACP's statement that the duty to the individual patient should always be considered primary when it is in conflict with other obligations.

NURSING AND PROFESSIONALISM

Nursing, also the heir of a long tradition, has been considered a healthcare profession for most of this century, and meets all of the criteria for a profession discussed above. It too has professional ethics codes which reinforce the traditional primary commitment to the health and well-being of the patient for whom the nurse cares. But like the engineer, and unlike the physician, the nurse has never had the autonomy or control over the conditions of professional practice which have characterized the role of the physician. The majority of nurses have always been, and most still are, employees, either of physicians or of hospitals, and are constrained by their professional codes, as well as by organizational structures, to implementing and supporting the work of the physician, who has primary legal and professional responsibility for diagnosis and medical treatment.

Prior to the 1970s the American Nurses Association (ANA) advocated a traditionalist position, purportedly based on the nineteenth-century philosophy of Florence Nightingale. This position held that the nurse had a primary obligation to her patient and that the best way for this obligation to be fulfilled was via cooperation with physicians. This position became controversial for many reasons, including increasing professionalization and the perception that, because of the sexism of society and the gender distribution across the two professions (in 1963, fully 98 percent of nurses were female and 96 percent of physicians were male), "cooperation" with doctors was often manifested as subordination. The popular notion that Nightingale had advocated obedience to the physician as the primary obligation of the nurse was particularly problematic; in fact, she envisaged something more like a sharp division of labor. She recommended the establishment of nursing as an autonomous but parallel profession to medicine, having control of patient care, as contrasted with patient medical treatment.

In the mid-1970s the ANA took a major step that is reflected in its 1976 Code for Nurses. The ANA promulgate changed this code to the concept of "client advocacy" as the guiding professional precept for nurses. Client advocacy emphasizes the autonomy and rights of the client(patient), and models the nurse/client relationship as a freely negotiated and expressed contract between the professional nurse and the "client," in contrast to the previous emphasis on care and beneficence of the nurse and her fiduciary duty to the "patient" (Husted & Husted, 1991). One important aspect of this reformulation for the self-understanding of nursing was that it recognized the extent to which the nurse-patient relationship was a separate and distinguishable set of obligations and professional services, rather than a transparent mediation or simple extension of the physician-patient relationship.

Although this position was generally embraced by academic nursing, many practicing nurses thought it undervalued the fiduciary duty of the nurse to the patient, and by terming the patient a "client" suggested a less appropriate model for nursing care. Recently, more academic nurses have been advocating a change back toward the service-oriented position of nursing prior to the mid-1970s. Sally Gadow, for instance, has written that care is the supreme covenant between the nurse and the patient and that care is the moral basis for the nurse-patient relationship. She does not equate this position with any degree of subservience to physician, but believes it better expresses the parallel between the two professions. Further, the idea of a "covenant" acknowledges a professional responsibility that goes beyond a negotiated contractual relationship between the nurse and the client, which she believes actually destroys the idea of the nurse as a professional (Gadow, 1988).

TRADITIONALISM, COMMUNITARIANISM, OR A NEW PROFESSIONAL ETHICS FORMULATION?

The institutionalization of health care into organizations has raised a number of issues for healthcare professionals, issues to which we have alluded in previous sections. One important question is whether it is really necessary to maintain medicine and other related aspects of health care as traditional professions, or if the traditionalist approach to professional ethics must be abandoned completely. Some have suggested that a compromise is possible, and one such compromise could be termed a "communitarian" approach to professional ethics.

The AMA addressed this issue in 1996, by sponsoring a symposium in Philadelphia entitled, "Ethics and American Medicine: History, Change and Challenge." At this meeting a number of prominent physicians and other professionals spoke about ethical issues in medicine with a particular emphasis on an ethical vision for the medical profession for the future. Although the symposium focused on the physician, we will extrapolate their concerns for all healthcare professionals.

An important focus of discussion were the two basic fundamental positions concerning the professionalism of medicine today: one which we call the traditionalist position and the other, the communitarian position. The traditionalist position, represented by Edmund Pellegrino, M.D., of the Center for Clinical Bioethics at Georgetown University and Mark Siegler, M.D., director of the MacLean Center for Clinical Medical Ethics at the University of Chicago, calls for a return to or at least a reinvigoration of the traditional view of medicine. In this view, medicine is a calling of the highest human dimension, a calling that can only thrive in a climate where the healthcare professional sees himself and is seen by others to have a primary fiduciary obligation to his particular patient. This obligation should supersede all others and must be present within the context of the professional-patient relationship (Journal of the American Medical Association, 1997).

Those who advocate a traditionalist position see issues such as the financial aspects of health care as distractions that ideally should have little to do with the obligations of the healthcare professional toward her patients and the work that she does within this context. They recognize that today's healthcare system requires professionals to attend to their obligations to the community and to others who are not her patients (public health issues, medical research issues, etc). However, they believe that professional obligations are hierarchically ordered, and that the obligation to the patient should be primary. When there is a conflict with other obligations, it always must take precedence.

Proponents of the communitarian position at the AMA symposium included Alexander Capron, L.L.B., codirector of the Pacific Center for Health Policy and Ethics at the University of Southern California, and Robert Veatch, Ph.D., professor of medical ethics at the Kennedy Institute of Ethics, Georgetown University. Troyen Brennan, a clinical ethicist at Harvard University School of Medicine, also supports the position. Capron, who calls for the creation of a "postmodern medical ethics" best states the communitarian position:

1. Uncertainty itself is a feature of ethics.
2. Technical expertise does not justify control of medical ethics by physicians alone.
3. The core value in traditional medical ethics—making the interests of patients paramount—must still shape the content of the new ethics, but new codes must be developed that depend on clear ideas about the purposes of the profession, that is, the ends of medicine.

Capron concludes, "The challenges to medicine today—the replacement of a profession guided by ethics by a business guided by competition —, the acquiescence of physicians [and other healthcare professionals] to demands of payers and patients, the barriers to access for a large part of the public—make necessary the movement to a new ethics, in which no one party asserts sole control but also in which the medical profession plays an essential role dealing with issues at the heart of modern health care and not simply filigrees around the borders" (*Journal of the American Medical Association*, 1997, p. 1267).

Veatch believes that "society will be the authority that controls and shapes medical ethics" (*Journal of the American Medical Association*, 1997, p. 1266). Brennan has stated this position even more directly: "Traditional ethical notions must be modified because doctors [and other healthcare professionals] can no longer say, 'the patient comes first' for they must also consider the hospital, the group practice, and the publicly approved reimbursement scheme" (Abrams, 1997, p. 1123).

To draw a contrast between the two positions, we may have to exaggerate and possibly distort the actual positions of the proponents. However, the contrast may help us draw some distinctions that will be useful as we consider professional ethics in the contemporary situation.

The traditionalist position holds that:

1. Medicine is a monolithic ethical enterprise, defined in terms of the achievement of one dominating good, the end or defining goal of medicine.
2. The professional obligation is to specify the end of medicine; to determine the best means to that end; and to act accordingly. (A corollary to this premise is that it is the physician's right, and the physician's alone, to make that judgment.)
3. Any other obligations the physician has (and there are many, including the obligation to provide for his own survival) must be subordinated to the dominant end of medicine.

4. That dominant end is the physician-patient relationship, which commits the physician to benefiting and not harming the patient, to being an active advocate for the care and well-being of the patient.

The communitarian position challenges each of those premises:

1. Medicine is not a monolithic ethical enterprise; it must acknowledge a plurality of possible ends, purposes, or goals which medicine serves, and adjudicate between them depending upon the circumstances.
2. The necessary corollary of the plurality claim would be the conclusion that ethics in medicine, like the art of medicine itself, must allow for some degree of uncertainty.
3. Medicine is not a purely individualistic enterprise; others have a say in the decisions fundamental to medical practice, which may include some say in what treatments are to be allowed. (In practice, physicians have long since moved to the notion of team medicine and patient rights, both of which are qualifications of "sole control by physicians alone.")
4. The physician has obligations not only to his patient but to the class of patients, and thus to principles of distributive justice, which affect medical care; and obligations of stewardship to the resources entrusted to him.

PROFESSIONAL ETHICS AND THE ETHICAL CLIMATE OF HCOS

How do the divergent ideas about the ethical ideals of health care affect the operation of the HCO? Does it really matter whether one adheres to a traditionalist or communitarian perspective? More importantly for our purposes, how do these professional perspectives affect the development and functioning of an organization ethics program in the HCO? These issues are some of the most important affecting the likelihood of success of the organization ethics program in its primary function of developing and maintaining a consistent ethical climate for the HCO.

The traditionalist position has much to commend it. It is the ideal most healthcare professionals aspire to and most patients rely upon as the basis for medicine. But, in its pure form such a position is essentially impossible to maintain. Under contemporary conditions, professional organizations that profess commitment to an unmodified traditionalist position would only encourage the popular suspicion of their motives. This is because the idealized image of the caregiver as a professional totally dedicated to the wants and needs of his patient is not generally true. George Lundberg, former editor of the *Journal of the American Medical Association* has argued, "From antiquity, medicine has been and continues to be both a business and a profession. Physicians are, by definition, both entrepreneurs and professionals. The issue, then is one of balance—I believe there are two coexisting components-business and professionalism. At the extreme end of the business side are the 'money grubbers.' At the extreme end of professionalism are the 'altruistic missionaries.' Most physicians are more nearly in the center of the curve" (Lundberg, 1997, p. 1704).

Lundberg believes that this double "end of medicine" should be openly acknowledged. He does not wish to abandon the ideal of sole control over practice conditions and patient treatment, however; instead, he would like to see the threat of alternative values—especially the lure of personal welfare—eliminated. He recommends that physicians and other healthcare professionals demand that their professional codes include stricter requirements for self-governance, self-determination and self-policing and that members of the profession should then perform in good faith by following their stringent ethical code.

Lundberg's diagnosis is accurate, but his prescription, if not impossible, is nearly so, for several reasons. In the first place, professionalism has always recommended a very similar prescription, but has a bad track record of implementing it. A claim that "this time we'll stick to it" is likely to be met with public skepticism. In the second place, even if it would work, we see little movement by any recognized medical group in the direction Lundberg advocates. Further, even if the professional organizations did get behind a move to revitalize the traditionalist approach, it is unlikely that the current changes in the healthcare system will move toward the validation of any such single-minded and inflexible self-determining, self-directed, self-policing organization of physicians.

Finally, there is a real question whether the recommendations of the traditionalist position are even remotely possible, much less desirable. If one adheres to a purely traditionalist perspective, the physician in particular, will be expected to act always as an advocate for the needs, and perhaps even the desires, of her individual patient while in the HCO. When all possible interventions that might have benefit are not available for all patients, this position can, and often will, set one of the physician's patients against another of the same physician's patients, one physician against another, or one physician against other professionals and managers within the HCO. Unless the persons with final decision-making authority decide that the HCO will respond positively to all requests from physicians concerning treatment for their individual patients—an option that is now, and indeed probably has always been, economically unfeasible, the purely traditionalist perspective will not function adequately. An effort to adhere to this point of view will, in all likelihood, destroy any effort to develop a consistent ethical climate for the HCO. The HCO cannot realistically respond positively to all physician requests and remain in operation, and to fulfill its obligations to its patient community, it obviously must continue to operate.

This discouraging litany suggests that some version of what we have called the communitarian perspective is the best hope for accommodating professional ethics to institutional medicine, and the only perspective that will fit within the context of developing an ethical climate for the modern HCO. If we try to think about a model for professional ethics that does not require the absolute control over the conditions of practice that the traditionalist model recommends and that physicians earlier in the century might have approximated, but can no longer claim; a model which acknowledges a cooperative and reciprocal relation not only to the individuals within its realm of practice and to other collaborating healthcare professionals, but also to the society which has institutionalized professions for specific purposes (which are subject to revisitation at all points)—we will have a model much closer to the communitarian than the traditionalist positions we have sketched. We will certainly have a model that is closer to the actual beliefs and practices of the professions, and one which will allow us to shape our understanding of the values of medicine to accommodate changing conditions.

This perspective is much like traditional stakeholder theory for business ethics. It allows for consideration of the positions of all whom have an interest in the issue at hand. It involves an analysis of who most affects or is affected by the issue at hand within the context of the organization, and requires an analysis of the relative strengths of the claims of those involved. The difficulty is, as we argued in Chapter 4, if one or more of these stakeholder claims seem stronger than the concerns of the individual patient, then that claim takes precedence. This perspective will not allow for ignoring or downplaying any legitimate obligation whether at the level of the individual patient, the HCO, a managed care organization, a group practice, or the community. In the latter part of Chapter 4 we developed a more complex stakeholder model for HCOs that gave priority to patients and patient populations. But that model also presents difficulties in determining when the patient has an absolute claim and therefore does not fit so neatly into a communitarian perspective as it is currently framed.

Furthermore, those who support the communitarian perspective have forgotten or neglected one important factor in modern health care. Patients want a healthcare professional they can trust to be an advocate for their interests, not one who negotiates with them while considering other issues such as the appropriate allocation of resources, or the relative merits of their claim on a certain scarce treatment as compared with another's claim. Whether our society is now or will ever be ready to change its perception of what a good healthcare professional should be, is open to question, however, there is little indication at present that a change in this perception is likely.

One positive note—we as a society have already addressed this particular issue in a specific area using the methods that have been developed by the United Network for Organ Sharing (UNOS) for the selection of recipients of scarce organs. Under UNOS guidelines, physicians are expected to continue to advocate for their individual patients while at the same time the physician and her patient are expected to understand that another may have a greater claim on the available organ under UNOS guidelines. This mechanism has gone relatively smoothly because most see it as the fairest way possible to solve a difficult problem.

Unfortunately, there have been few attempts to develop a practical approach to the healthcare professional's ethics in the modern HCO. Attention to this very important area is mandatory if an organization ethics program is to have a chance to be more than an on-paper response to accreditation requirements and negative governmental attention. How can we integrate the professional ethics of the healthcare professionals into the organization ethics program in such a way that the integrity of the professions is maintained while allowing for unique decision making in a specific HCO?

We agree with the traditionalist position that the healthcare professional must remain an advocate for his patient's interests. However, this may not mean exactly what some have understood it to mean in the past. The healthcare professional has never been considered either by himself or by his patient to be devoted only to advocacy for one patient. He has had to divide his time based on competing needs of a number of patients as well as personal and family needs. He has been expected to use his specialized knowledge to help the patient understand the limitations of specific interventions as well as the limitations (including financial constraints), imposed from the outside. As long as the healthcare professional has been open and completely honest with the patient, there has been little difficulty with this type of advocacy.

Newer ways of approaching the delivery and financing of health care have added new and different considerations into this decision-making and advocacy equation, but they have not changed the outline of the equation itself. The healthcare professional is still expected to advocate for her patients within the context of the medical, financial, and administrative situation, and as long as this context is fully understood by patients, trust remains and the professional truly continues as the patient's trusted advocate.

The code of any of the recognized professional organizations could be the basis for the ethics of medicine and health care in the future, but revisions will be necessary if these codes are to function adequately in the healthcare organization of today and tomorrow. The code and principles of the Council of Medical Specialty Societies (CMSS) illustrates a model that maintains traditional obligations while at the same time allows for the development of a consistent ethical climate in a HCO, an ethical climate that can support and strengthen professional ethics.

In April 1998, the Council of Medical Specialty Societies (CMSS), a professional organization representing a number of groups of medical specialists, released a "Consensus Statement on the Ethic of Medicine," in which it advanced its framework for the ethical base for health care today. The preamble to this consensus statement begins as follows: "The practice of medicine is rooted in a covenant of trust among patients, physicians and society. The ethic of medicine must seek to balance the physician's responsibility to each patient and the professional collective obligation to all who need medical care" (Council of Medical Specialty Societies, 1998, p. 2). Notice the recognition of the possible conflicts of commitment and the accompanying conflicting obligations for healthcare professionals in this statement. This particular set of ethical principles is based on a traditional character-based perspective, but recognizes the importance of the issues embedded in the U.S. healthcare system. The code for CMSS was developed for physicians, but it is eminently suitable as a possible code for most healthcare professionals in HCOs, as our notations in brackets indicate. Particular principles advanced by the CMSS include:

1. "The physician's [nurse's, and other healthcare professional's] primary inviolate role is as an active advocate for each patient's care and well being."
2. "The physician's [nurse's, and other healthcare professional's] duty of patient advocacy should not be altered by the system of healthcare delivery in which the physician practices."
3. "Physicians [nurses, and other healthcare professionals] should resolve conflicts of interest in a fashion that gives primacy to the patient's interests."
4. "Physicians [nurses, and other healthcare professionals] should provide knowledgeable input into organizational decisions on the allocation of medical resources and the process of healthcare delivery."
5. "Physicians [nurses, and other healthcare professionals] have a responsibility to serve the healthcare needs of all members of society."
6. "Physicians [nurses, and other healthcare professionals] have an ethical obligation to participate in the formation of healthcare policy."
7. "Physicians [nurses, and other healthcare professionals] have an ethical obligation to preserve and protect the trust bestowed on them by society" pp. 2–8).

This code comes closest to presenting a workable model of the obligations of healthcare professionals in today's healthcare system. In doing so, its principles and guidelines reinvigorate some degree of professional power in healthcare organizations.

How should a developing organization ethics program approach the task of integrating the healthcare professional defined by the CMSS into the ethical climate of the HCO? First, the HCO's organization ethics program should recognize that all healthcare professionals will maintain some type of consistent external (to the HCO) professional mandate defining, in general terms, the obligations of the professional and that these general obligations will form the parameters for the activities and duties of the physician in the HCO. Then, during its development, the organization ethics program should initiate and support conversations with professional groups with the expressed purpose of developing an appropriate local code of behavior for professional groups and integrating that code into the ethical climate of the HCO. Specific professional groups should develop their particular codes while in conversation with the other departments and groups affected by the code and with the group responsible for the organization ethics program. External professional mandates will have set the parameters within which the more specific code for the HCO is developed. This mechanism allows for local control of the specific details of the professionals' ethics while maintaining broad general mandates for all members of the profession. This method encourages conversation, it should lead to better understanding, and it does not dismiss one of the most important traditional aspects of professional ethics, that of maintaining advocacy for the patient.

The major objection to this idea is that it appears to put more power back into the hands of professionals. This may or may not be true. If the core mission of an HCO is patient and population health care, and we suggested in Chapter 1 that this should be the case, then this mission coincides with codes of healthcare professionals. Thus the mission of the organization supports and reinforces the priorities of professional mandates. If patient and population health care is not prioritized as the core mission of the HCO, then one wonders how it can be called a *healthcare* organization; and questions about its implicit social contract would surely be at issue. The coincidence of HCO mission and professional mandates does not solve all conflicts of interest or conflicts of commitment nor does it address a number of important ethical issues in the delivery of healthcare. However, it eliminates one source of confusion, it retains the ideal of professionalism that society expects in its professionals and its healthcare organizations, and the patient, the professional, the HCO, and society should all benefit.

6

The Relationship of Social Climate
to the Historical Development of the Healthcare
Organization and Its Ethical Climate

Our healthcare organizations owe much of their form and function, as well as their publicly perceived mission, to their particular history in the United States and the social, economic, and political conditions under which they operate.

The organization of health and hospital services has always reflected changing societal values and interests. These societal interests shape the ethical climate within which healthcare organizations operate. They help determine how their income is derived, who has the power to affect their direction and everyday operation, and how their mission is perceived and judged. The changing relationships within an HCO itself (involving the board of directors, administrators, medical staff, other clinical staff, ancillary staff, hourly employees, and, most importantly, patients) as well as the relationships between individuals or groups representing the HCO and interested persons outside the organization are also important factors when attempting to analyze its ethical climate.

The idea of ethical climate has a long history in organization theory. As an internal characteristic, it stems from the perception of its ethical structure by members of the organization. The ethical structure of an organization consists of the values, principles, rules, purposes, and ideals that characterize its operation and are manifested in its practices and procedures. The ranking of values and their salience or relative invisibility are part of the institutional structure. While it has become increasingly common to express the goals, values, and ethical expectations in explicit ethics statements, values statements, or mission statements, these modern codifications are just the most recent form of understanding normative expectations, which have existed as long as there have been institutions to serve specific social purposes. The *internal* ethical climate is the expressed understanding of people within the organization as to how well the organization lives up to its purposes and social role, its expressed values, what values they see their jobs as fulfilling, and the tasks and standards that characterize their role in the institution (Schneider, 1975, pp. 460–461). In the business literature, the organizational (or ethical) climate is primarily derived from internal characteristics, such as how an organization is seen by its constituent members, the priorities given to various values, and the congruence with member expectations. Thus, it is defined by the shared perception of how ethical issues should be addressed and what constitutes ethical behavior (Joseph & Deshpande, 1997, p. 77).

There is an external, or environmental, component as well to ethical climate, as we will be using the term in this and the next chapter. The content of the ethical structure is seldom the arbitrary creation of the organization itself; instead, it is the internalization into the institution's self-understanding of what is expected of the institution by the society of which it is a functioning component. Those expectations, the role in the society which an organization is expected to play, constitute the *external* ethical climate, and to the extent they are internalized become the ethical structure. In this chapter we will look in some detail at what American society's expectations of the HCO have been at various stages of its development. Consonant with Figure 2.1, this book considers organizations as midlevel ethical agents. Organizations have a part to play in the larger society of which they are components, as well as having responsibilities to the individuals who constitute them or are affected by their operations. As we use the term, the ethical climate of an organization incorporates not only the descriptions and beliefs about its values and priorities of those who fill roles in the organization, but also is responding to the needs and demands of the larger society which has designated organizations to fulfill certain roles in that society. Those demands affect and inform its ethical structure. Thus an HCO *has* an internal ethical climate; but it also operates *within*, and is to some extent determined by, an external ethical climate.

As we will see in this and the next chapter, social construction of the role of the HCO has changed since the early days of the republic and is even now in the throes of another radical transformation. In order to understand the ethical climate of the HCO, and in order to be able to suggest mechanisms to positively affect the internal ethical climate, it will be useful to explore the history of the HCO and the changing expectations of it, both by its internal constituents and by the larger society. This chapter then represents a study of the external ethical climate—shifts in the demands on HCO and the needs they serve that in turn alter the roles of individuals within the institution.

The ethical climate of an organization, as we are using the term in this book, is a relation between the *expectations* of an organization (its expectations of itself and the expectations others have of it) and its *accomplishments*. If the decisions, actions, and projects of an organization, and the results of those actions, are consonant with what is expected of it, we judged it to have a good, that is, a positive, ethical climate. If there is a wide disparity between expectations and results, there is reason to question the ethical soundness of the organization, to ascribe to it a negative ethical climate. The language we apply to the latter organization—*bad*, *unsound*—suggests an analogy between the ethical climate of an organization and the health of an individual. Like our own health, the ethical climate of our organizations should be good. If it isn't, that perception of disparity between expectation and achievement represents a problem that needs to be addressed. As members of our society, as agents of, employees of, and contributors to HCOs, and as potential recipients of the care they provide, we want and need ethically positive, ethically healthy, HCOs.

A disparity between the expectations of an organization and its accomplishments can have a variety of causes, and if we are to take seriously organization ethics as a project for HCOs it behooves us to be as clear as we can about ways in which ethical climate can be less than ideal. There are expectations of the HCO from all three levels: the individual level, from other organizations, as well as from the larger society. For instance, society can have unrealistic, unclear, or contradictory expectations of an HCO. Particularly in times of transition, we may find that while the conditions under which an organization operates have changed, the expectations others have of them have not; or vice versa. The changes over time in the role of the HCO depicted in our historical sketch represent a reciprocal accommodation between the HCO and the changing expectations of society.

An organization can have unclear, contradictory, or unrealistic expectations of itself as well. Any of those qualifications make it likely that it will fail to meet its own expectations or the expectations of its constituent members, with consequent disappointment, demoralization, and low morale. It is of course possible to have perfectly consistent, realistic, and clear expectations of your organization and still fail to meet them; there are bad organizations, as well as bad luck. But failure to meet impossible expectations is not a moral failure.

In this chapter we consider the history and the changing relationships of various constituencies of the HCO both in terms of their effects on the HCO and also in terms of the values that influenced the development and operation of HCOs since the late eighteenth century. We will also try to extrapolate from historical data what the ethical expectations were for HCOs in the past, the external ethical climate which determined their ethical structure, and what this meant to the part they played in their communities and in society.

We will consider the HCO's history in three time periods: from the early days of the republic to the Civil War, from the Civil War to the end of World War II, and from the immediate postwar period to the failure of the Clinton "Health Security Plan" (see Chapter 7) and its attempt to reorganize the U.S. healthcare system (in about 1994). Each of these periods encompasses a time of relative stability in the larger conceptualization of what an HCO should be, and in the major influences on the HCO. Major changes in the internal and external social and political influences on the HCO occurred as the next period and its time of relative stability was supplanting each of the previous historical periods.

The first period is characterized by the strong paternalism of boards of trustees based on religious and social values that expressed a sense of charitable obligation to the poor. The second period saw the overriding influence of trustees being replaced by a "medicalized" paternalism, with the power vested chiefly in physicians. The third period represented the increasing influence of insurance companies and the federal government, leading to a concentration of power in the administrative offices of the HCO. All of the changes had a major effect on the ethical climate of the HCO of the time period. Internally changing values, methods of operation, and shifts of power among internal HCO stakeholders manifested these changes. The period from 1994 to the present will be discussed in the next chapter, which looks at the healthcare system of today and how the changes in the external ethical climate affected the internal ethical climate of the HCO.

In discussing the historical development of the HCO and the concomitant development of its internal ethical climate we will concentrate mainly on the hospital as the important HCO with some attention to the forerunner of the modern nursing home, the almshouse, in the initial period. In Appendix 5 we have included a discussion of the rapid development of modern nursing homes and their subsequent problems, both of which have had a profound effect on the ability of a nursing home to support a consistent internal ethical climate.

AMERICAN HOSPITALS: EIGHTEENTH CENTURY TO THE CIVIL WAR

If we describe hospitals as institutions dedicated exclusively to inpatient care of the sick, in 1800 there were only two in the United States, the Pennsylvania Hospital and New York Hospital. The Pennsylvania Hospital was founded in Philadelphia in 1752; New York Hospital opened its doors in the 1790s. The third great hospital of this period, Massachusetts General Hospital, did not begin operations until 1821. These hospitals from their inception were staffed by the elite physicians of the time, but had been developed and were actively supported by philanthropists who decided on all aspects of the operation of the hospitals, including the values that supported their mission. The decision-making authority of these philanthropists emanated from their role as members of the boards of trustees of these hospitals.

These major hospitals quickly became a source of pride for their communities. They became the site of the beginnings of medical education in this country and attracted prominent physicians to their staffs. Their patients were either the working poor, or those who were considered of higher station and had had an unexpected tragedy resulting in what was expected to be a temporary condition. These patients were believed to be deserving of good care and help since they were expected to return to being, or to become, productive citizens. Perhaps more importantly, these patients were considered deserving because they had not deviated appreciably from the prevailing moral norms of the time.

During the first half of the nineteenth century one or more large hospitals were established in most major cities. The philanthropic boards of trustees who were involved in developing these large city hospitals saw the development and operation of these hospitals as an important way to fulfill their duty to care for the deserving poor. Notice the distinction between the deserving poor, which the trustees considered as the appropriate focus for the development of these institutions, and the undeserving poor, who at that time were relegated to institutions set aside for less desirable citizens, the almshouses.

The trustees of these large hospitals took a paternalistic but generally impersonal view of the patients in their institutions. They developed and maintained formal admissions procedures and a hierarchical administrative structure. There were, however, some real differences among these institutions. Many of the first hospitals were founded and supported by specific religious denominations and emphasized providing moral, as well as physical and medical, succor for their patients. Some were designated as "women's hospitals" and provided food and shelter particularly for pregnant women (mainly unwed mothers) for prolonged periods. "Children's hospitals" tended to resemble orphanages. In this sense, these large hospitals reflected the idiosyncratic goals of their founders or the particular needs of their clientele rather than conforming to any shared social definition of what a hospital should be (Rosner, 1982, p. 2).

Patients in all of these large hospitals continued to be mainly those who had too few resources to be treated at home, which was by far the preferred method for recovering from an illness or accident. Respectable persons with adequate means were treated at home, since there was little effective treatment available at that time, and what was available could just as easily be given at home by a visiting physician or nurse. Also the hospitals, even the premiere ones, were dangerous places. Patients with infectious diseases of all types were placed together in wards, and cross-infection was common. All in all, staying at home for medical treatment, if you could afford it, was not just a sign of social importance, but was an exceedingly wise course of action. No person of property would have been found in even the respected large city hospitals unless stricken with insanity or taken severely ill or the victim of an accident away from his home.

In spite of the early development of the large city hospitals, most medicine in the nineteenth century was focused on small communities and narrow personal contacts. Most Americans lived in isolated rural villages and towns. Even the cities of the time were much more collections of neighborhoods with their own culture and values than large homogeneous entities. Medical practice was a part of this culture, and physicians treated patients in their community at their homes. Family practitioners constituted the bulk of the profession and lived within the communities they served, providing healthcare services from their own home or from an office adjacent to their home. Hospitals for these communities, when available, were small, local, and dependent on local charity, religious sponsorship, or governmental largess for operating expenses.

By the early to mid nineteenth century, a number of these smaller local hospitals had been formed, differing in size, medical orientation, type and level of services, financial support, and religious or ethnic orientation. The large public and charity hospitals in the bigger cities continued to be looked upon as adjuncts to local hospitals and almshouses and served those who could not be accommodated in the small local facilities. The local hospitals sent the "unworthy" poor, alcoholics, and criminals to the large public hospitals and almshouses while attempting to serve the deserving poor and the working class from their community.

Unlike modern hospitals, these small nineteenth-century community hospitals were not solely medical facilities but facilities that also occasionally provided for other needs, including food and shelter. Need for hospital admission was frequently more dependent on a social condition, such as family situation or economic status, rather than a medical problem. Servants, particularly, had no place else to go when unable to perform their duties due to illness or injury. The hospital was a healthcare facility, a social service, and an agent of social control. It supported cultural consistency even in the face of what at other times might have been major upheavals; times of significant immigration and economic uncertainty. Hospitals of the time with a religious affiliation had an additional role, the role of evangelism to their nonbelieving patients, and this role was taken quite seriously.

Unlike hospitals, almshouses in towns and cities from the late eighteenth century to the twentieth century provided custodial and sometimes medical care for the socially undesirable and destitute. The almshouse, if not always a site for care, was at least a place to reside while recovering from an illness. Almshouses were also residences for the indigent and often for the mentally ill, although the latter were at a later date afforded a specific type of almshouse, the asylum. The almshouse was seen mainly as an appropriate social structure for separating the ill, the destitute, the permanently incapacitated, and other dependent persons considered to be undesirable and undeserving, from the rest of society. In larger cities the almshouse supported a large number of sick individuals who had the potential to recover and return to society, so some attempt was often made to segregate the ill from the more permanent residents of the almshouse. Some almshouses supported physician's visits to the sick as often as three or four times a week.

Throughout this entire period the average physician's practice was chiefly home-based. Highly renowned physicians were often associated with the more prominent hospitals, but even they maintained an independent home-based practice and were subject to the rules imposed by the ruling board of trustees while attending in the hospital. The early hospital offered the ambitious physician a chance to improve his skills and learning. However, the fact that society suspected that the physician might learn at the expense of his patients prevented the physician from having much say in the governance of the hospital. Practice at a prestigious hospital did offer the physician a chance to increase his prestige within the local community and advance his interests in this and other ways (Starr, 1982, p. 152).

Although morally upright, patients occupying beds in the hospitals were thought to need moral limits. Not only did this attitude apply to patients, but it was also extended to those who worked in the institutions including nurses, house staff, and other attendants (Rosenberg, 1987, p. 35). For this and other more practical reasons, order was a high priority in these hospitals, especially important to the trustees who ran the hospitals. Although such rules were not always consistently enforced, the intention that there be strict routines for all activities and decision making within these institutions was completely paternalistic. Convalescent and ambulatory patients worked while in the institution and laboring expectant mothers were expected to lend a hand when able.

The administrator of the hospital, the superintendent (and his wife, who was expected to oversee such "ladies'" functions as doing the laundry) was drawn from the community ranks. Trustees expected the superintendent to serve as father figure and so expected him and his family to live within the hospital. No experience or medical training was required or expected. The superintendent was there to translate the mandates of the board into practical actions. He was expected to possess the virtues of prudence, responsibility, and piety (Rosenberg, 1987, p. 42).

An important aspect of the superintendent's job was to supervise the nursing activities in his institution. Nurses at this time were not yet considered professionals. They were trained on the job to the extent necessary to fulfill the needed functions. Wages for nursing positions were low, and nursing became a haven for those who could secure no better-paying position (Flanagan, 1976).

We have said that the internal ethical climate of an HCO is a function of the perception of the ethical structure of the organization, which is itself influenced by the expectations of the society of what that institution should do—the external ethical climate within which it operates. It is the individual or group within the organization which has the most power, and thus greatest influence, upon the HCO that determines that ethical structure.

The governing board of trustees, even if not always the source of financial support, determined the values and mission of the HCOs of this period. Since hospital board members were prominent citizens, and particularly since many of them supported the hospital financially, there was seldom any questioning of their direction of the institution. It was the board's expectations of the institution that determined the organization's expectations of itself. Hospitals of the time did focus on medical care and saw as their mission a mandate to advance the health of their patients by treating them according to the best knowledge of the time, and the role of the physician was to advance that part of the mission. But in addition to this focus on medical care was the ideal of returning these patients to their proper station in life and enhancing their ability to live moral lives. Medical treatment in these facilities accompanied the overt association of the hospital with a particular moral stance, often religiously based. The hospital was expected to enhance the religious and social ability of its patients, as well as to improve their health, and it was the institution's success or failure at this double task which determined its value to the community and strongly influenced its ethical climate. It was not a climate where the specific rights of individual patients had much of an impact on the goals or methods for treatment. Insofar as the hospital was paternalistic, it was not the physicians, but the board, which determined the moral stance of the institution. The ethical structure of one hospital could differ from that of another in minor ways, but all tended to be broadly based on the ideal of compassion for the deserving ill, with minimal attention to those considered less deserving.

The larger hospitals of the day, like their later successors, were also the site of research and education, and they were useful to the physicians of the day for those reasons. Patients were useful as research subjects and educational material, and their contribution to those objectives was assumed when they were admitted to the hospital. Since the more influential members of the society were unlikely to be hospital patients, being cared for instead in the comfort and privacy of their own homes, there was little controversy within the hospital, or within the society which supported it, about the appropriateness of this expectation.

The social expectations, and thus the ethical structure, of the almshouse of this period was even less salubrious. The almshouse was looked upon as a necessary demonstration of Christian ideals and was therefore supported mainly by churches and the religious community. Christian charity required minimum sustenance but certainly not more than this. Although possibly slightly better than being abandoned in the streets, the atmosphere of the average almshouse must have been grim and, for most of its residents, hopeless. Medical care as a part of the duty of almshouses was minimal and often consisted only of substandard food and a place to sleep. Here, too, governance was totally autocratic with the rules coming from the responsible parties, including the staff. The ethical climate of the almshouse, in many cases, more closely resembled that of a prison than any other type of institution.

AMERICAN HOSPITALS: CIVIL WAR TO WORLD WAR II

The period from the Civil War to World War II was a period of significant change in that it saw the professionalization of the American hospital. From the immediate period following the Civil War to the 1940s, the tendency was for both the large and small hospitals to become less idiosyncratic, leading to the development of acute-care facilities similar to those we are familiar with today. During this period medical care improved greatly, enhancing the prominence and power of the physician in the hospital. By the end of this period, most U.S. hospitals had uniform admissions procedures, a hierarchical administrative structure, and income derived chiefly from patient payments.

During the Civil War over one million men were treated in Union hospitals. Remarkably, the death rate was less than 10 percent. Specific treatment modalities in the Civil War were not significantly advanced beyond those employed a century earlier (with the major exception of anesthesia), yet this dramatically low death rate occurred through simple changes in diet, cleanliness, warmth, and ventilation. There had been some obvious advances in battlefield surgical technique, but making the hospital an effective and efficient place for healing, and ultimately for returning soldiers to military duty, was the major advance, an advance which has influenced important aspects of the acute-care hospital even today. The seeds for these changes, which were so dramatically demonstrated during the Civil War, had been sown in the twenty years prior to the war by a number of hospital reformers, including Florence Nightingale (Flanagan, 1976). Acceleration of medical knowledge during this period, combined with implementation of medical advances (germ theory, antisepsis, better surgical techniques) following the Civil War, meant that physicians began acquiring skills based on technologies that could only be used effectively in an up-to-date and technologically well equipped hospital.

Because care was becoming more and more effective in the early twentieth century, all classes began to demand hospital admission. No longer was the hospital a manifestation of community stewardship and obligation to the poor, but it was increasingly seen as a resource for all individuals who were ill. As the perception spread that the hospital could be of benefit to all individuals, the number of hospitals throughout the country increased. In 1873 there were 178 hospitals in the United States; by 1923 this number had increased to 4,978 (Rosenberg, 1987, p. 341). Training schools for nurses, the major source of skilled labor for patient care, proliferated in the same period, marking the beginning of the professionalization of nursing.

These hospitals of the early twentieth century were in some ways very similar to their predecessors, but in other ways were totally different. The change from a charitable institution that provided services to the respectable poor to an organization that served individuals from the entire community had significant financial implications that reinforced and supported changes in the perceived role and mission of the hospital, as well as changes in the values upon which the role and mission depended. The hospital became less of an instrument for the community's obligation to its poorer citizens, and began to assume the stature of an important aspect of the community's day-to-day functioning. Factors influencing this change included medical advances such as those mentioned above, and changes in the training for physicians from an apprenticeship with one or more practitioners to association with a particular hospital. Just as importantly, political, economic, and social changes of the Progressive era such as increased immigration, new political realignments, and urban expansion all supported and advanced these changes.

Focus on the moral and social aspects of the patient diminished as concerns for the patient's medical condition increased. Effective control of the general hospital passed from lay groups to physicians, both because of the financial inability of the traditional donor class to maintain the expanding institution and the mounting assertiveness of physicians that accompanied medical professionalization of the hospital. This shift in control mirrored and was facilitated by the emergence of more-scientific attitudes toward values and society. Together these institutional and attitudinal shifts fostered the emergence of the hospital as a purely medical institution, with the patient as a clinical rather than a social or moral responsibility (Vogel, 1980, p. 3).

Financial solvency of the professionalized hospital demanded that patients drawn from the middle and upper classes pay for the services rendered, and such patients demanded better accommodations and services. The hospital became less dependent financially on the generosity of the members of the board of trustees and more dependent on physicians who admitted income-producing patients to the hospital. These important changes led to a two-tiered and sometimes multi-tiered system that treated paying patients much different from charity cases. This unequal treatment was recognized and accepted by most patients and strongly supported by the communities the hospitals served.

Although most everyday medical care was still located in patients' homes or in physicians' offices, surgical procedures were quickly shifting to the hospital. By the 1920s, surgery had become the most important aspect of hospital care (and also the most income producing) and was therefore the accepted key to hospital growth and financial solvency. This emphasis on surgery led to a continuing escalation of costs of hospital care as more and more technological interventions were needed for physicians and hospitals to remain up to date in the rapidly changing field of surgery. Increasing capital and operating costs required an ongoing quest for sources of income and endowment. Yet because of community expectations, few hospitals abandoned their historical mandate to care for the needy. Most boards retained the concept of stewardship developed during the previous period, which was particularly important in the religious foundations; and the physician of the day adhered to a professional ethic which demanded that patients be treated without regard to ability to pay.

By the early 1920s there was increasing influence of outside forces both within and beyond the community. Economic depression, political change, and a growing belief in medical expertise brought about new ways of doing things. New universal standards for hospitals determined the shape of healthcare organizations much more than the specific needs of the community or the patient population. Locally based charity facilities were being replaced by a more universal system built around the increasingly powerful medical profession and the hospital as representative of the state of the art of medical care in a particular community. The values of the community were still important to the board and were transmitted via the board to the administration and clinical staffs, but those values were changing as the expectations of the hospital changed. For any hospital to thrive it had to represent, within its particular community, a credible approximation of the best available medicine. Hospitals began to look like each other, to do the same things, and to focus on payment issues to remain in operation. Even though most remained nonprofit entities, efficient financial operation became much more important in this new competitive atmosphere. Even if a lay board of trustees remained titular head of hospital governance, many decisions were now made on the basis of the wants and needs of the physicians who staffed the hospital. Hospitals were doctors' institutions and the hospital was seen as a normal extension of the realm of influence and responsibility for physicians.

The increasing power of the physician within the hospital was not unchecked. Uneasy that controls were not being developed to monitor physicians' practices within the hospital, the American College of Surgeons* in 1919 introduced the "medical staff" as a quality-control element. The medical staff was defined as a self-directing entity within the hospital to which all physicians with admitting privileges belonged, and which set the standards for medical care in the hospital. Implementation of this concept within the hospital helped formalize and consolidate the transfer of power and prestige from the trustees to the physicians. This transfer is clearly expressed in such documents as hospital bylaws. By the mid-twentieth century ultimate responsibility for approval of medical staff bylaws was delegated to the board of trustees; but at the same time the bylaws often qualified that responsibility by stating that the governing body approval "shall not be unreasonably withheld" (Williams & Donnelly, 1982, p. 35).

The role of the administrator shifted as well. Operational responsibility within the HCO fluctuated among the physician, trustee, and administrator. Even though the physician controlled medical decision making in the hospital and had great influence on other decisions as well, tripartite responsibility for the operation of the hospital, with its potential for role confusion and conflict, continued into the 1930s and 1940s. The successful administrator of this time realized that success in managing the hospital depended less on technical ability and more on political ability to define his authority "both in opposition to and cooperation with medical men and lay trustees" (Rosenberg, 1987, p. 280). These astute administrators were the forerunners of the administrator of today.

---

*The American College of Surgeons is a scientific and educational association of surgeons that was founded in 1913 to improve the quality of care for the surgical patient by setting high standards for surgical education and practice. For more information visit the American College of Surgeons Web pages at http://www.facs.org/.

Nursing, by the early twentieth century, had begun to be recognized as an established and respected profession. There was a trained and disciplined nursing corps in many hospitals of the day, and many of those hospitals supported a training program for nurses. Standards of conduct were agreed to, and professional associations and journals were begun. In 1921, the American Nurses Association developed a statement on the ideals of the nursing profession (Flanagan, 1976, p. 81). This statement exhorted the nurse to gain the respect of physicians and to "endeavor to give such intelligent and skilled nursing service that she will be looked upon as a co-worker of the doctor in the whole field of health," as well as to "respect the physician as the person legally and professionally responsible for the medical and surgical treatment of the sick" (p. 90). The commitment of nurses to their patients was framed within the commitment of nurses to respect physicians, and the professionalization of nurses enhanced rather than undermined the growing stature of physicians within the hospital.

The change in the mission of the hospital from a charitable institution to a community wide resource for the care of the sick of all social strata meant that the physician became responsible for the well-being of a wider range of potential patients. Further, the physician was capable of a wider range of treatments as scientific and medical knowledge advanced, many of which could only be delivered through the hospital. Community expectations of the role of the hospital changed accordingly, and physicians were increasingly powerful within those institutions. Physicians set the educational and training standards for practice in a particular hospital. They developed their own quality control and quality-assurance techniques and determined what services the hospital offered. The administrative staff, which was generally responsible for the day-to-day operation of the hospital, had little to say about the medical interventions and specific care modalities, which were considered the responsibility of the medical staff.

The distinction between public and private care remained, even though both were more frequently provided within hospitals in this period. Public interest, and often public funding, were vested in the hospital, but the decisions concerning the use of the money were not public matters, but were left to others, mainly the physicians. The search for adequate funding to provide expected services for both paying patients and the poor became a dominant concern for the administrative staff and often for trustees and prominent members of the medical staff (Rosenberg, 1987, p. 345). But as institutional attention shifted from indigent care to community-wide care for mainly paying patients, the mission, the values upon which the mission was based, the structure of the HCO, and the roles and responsibilities of key stakeholder groups within the hospital changed.

If changes in social expectations produce changes in ethical structure and thus in ethical climate, the changes in the hospital from the time of the Civil War through the first half of the twentieth century were bound to have profound effects on the ethical climate of these institutions. Hospitals were expected to do more medically (and less morally) for a broader segment of the society. Hospitals were looking more alike, as they focused more on technological and medical issues, but were still predominantly local institutions, both in terms of their power base and in terms of their governance. The shift in power from the trustees to physicians accompanied a shift in the role of the hospital from a social institution with some (often ill-defined) medical responsibilities for a very limited constituency, the deserving indigent, to a medical institution with social responsibilities. The values of medicine became to a greater or lesser degree the values of the hospital. The professionalization of the nursing staff insured that these values were a part of the everyday work within the hospital.

Hospitals were also becoming more expensive. The importance of increasing sources of income necessitated changes that appealed to paying patients (private and semiprivate rooms; better meals; and other amenities, such as access to spiritual help and social work) and often led as well to the segregation of nonpaying patients to a "ward" status, which meant they were afforded few of the more costly innovations instituted to attract paying patients. The earlier tradition of hospitals as research and education institutions survived to some extent, in that these nonpaying patients were also expected by many to "volunteer" for research whereas the paying patients were not. A multitiered system of care was explicitly instituted within hospitals, and defended as socially appropriate, financially necessary, and compatible with the professional requirement that patients be treated without regard to ability to pay.

The physician was the prime mover in almost all hospitals of the time and it was the paternalism of the physician that was the most obvious force in determining what specific values were important in each hospital. But, in addition, the hospital had become a business, albeit a business with historical social obligations. How these sometimes conflicting values got sorted out in each individual hospital depended on the forcefulness of the physicians, the economic stress on the hospital, and the perceived social obligations as defined by the trustees and the administration. Suffice it to say that the patient had no real power to affect the operation of the hospital and that those in power decided on the appropriate values for the institution based on their perception of their professional and social obligations in regard to caring for the sick.

During this period there was little outside influence from government or other social or economic entities. The hospital was a place where the freedom of the physician was only questioned by another physician or occasionally by an administrator or board member if the issue in question was nonmedical. The patient's well-being was paramount and the physician determined what would enhance that well-being. It was only when the physician demanded costly interventions that threatened the survival of the institution that some trustees and administrators began to question this method of operating the institution. Medical expertise and power rapidly became as paternalistic and controlling as the social elitism it had replaced. Social and medical attitudes and practices reshaped the hospital; the hospital in turn influenced attitudes and practices beyond its walls as well as within. "The emergence of the modern hospital reflected a change in the kind of care the middle and upper class family offered its members. Removing birth, death, and often pain itself from the home led to changes in their significance; basic elements of human experience came to be redefined as medical events" (Vogel, 1980, p. 4).

These concerns ultimately led to changes occurring beyond the walls of the hospital that would profoundly change the hospital and its value system yet again. The most important of these changes was the institution of health insurance as a benefit of most jobs in the economy following the Second World War and the federal government's institution of Medicare and Medicaid in the mid 1960s.

What did those working within the hospital between the Civil War and World War II expect of their institutions? If times of transition are disruptive of ethical climate, it is fair to expect that there was a great deal of disruption of expectations as hospitals were transforming themselves decade by decade in that period. However, by the end of that period it is quite clear that professional values dominated the hospital, as the relationship of physician and hospital grew closer and closer. The tendency in the period was for more aspects of medical care to move into hospitals and out of homes, and expectations of what hospitals could do also were raised, as medical technology and research expanded. Standards for what constituted excellent medical care developed over the period, and were superimposed upon local community or denominational values. Hospitals began to look more alike, and to share an increasing acceptance of their medical over their social mission; indeed, improving the health of the community became a social mission in its own right. Class distinctions did not disappear from hospitals in this period, but they took a different form. Though earlier, economic status may have had some effect on whether you were in a hospital or elsewhere, now class distinctions moved within the hospital through a two-tiered system of paying versus charitable care. The physicians and nurses who worked within the hospitals were correspondingly expected to focus primarily on the medical needs of their patients, not their social worth, and to rely more and more on professional standards, which were consistent across institutions, for their values.

POST–WORLD WAR II HEALTHCARE SYSTEM

This is probably the period most familiar to our readers, and a period particularly difficult to treat in an abbreviated form. For the purposes of our enterprise, we would like to focus on the history of two important factors which have had the most impact on the contemporary HCO: the increasing influence of third-party payers (health insurers and the government), and the development of managed care organizations. As we all know, the confluence of these two factors is the major structural feature of the contemporary medical climate. In order to better understand this phenomenon, in the two following sections we will revisit the earlier eras as they affect the growth of the third-party payers. First we will look at the development of health insurance; then we will trace the history of the managed-care organization up to 1994.

Health insurance and government attention

Although this section deals with the HCO from the Second World War to the mid-1990s, some important changes that affected the ethical expectations of the HCO during this period had their beginnings in the 1920s and 1930s with the beginning of health insurance. The first real private health insurance in the United States began in 1929 at Baylor University in Texas, which initiated an insurance plan for schoolteachers in the area. Under this plan each teacher paid a small fee (fifty cents), for which the teacher received credit for a certain number of in-hospital days per year. Other hospitals in the Dallas area soon began offering similar plans. In 1932 in California a community-wide plan was developed under which participating hospitals in a given geographic area agreed to provide services to any of the plan's subscribers. Hospitals in other areas soon developed similar community-wide plans, which subsequently became known as Blue Cross plans. By 1938 the American Hospital Association began to promote noncompetitive community Blue Cross plans, and by 1940 the overall enrollment in these plans was about 6 million subscribers (Spencer, 1995).

Blue Cross plans covered only hospitalization and offered a single community-wide rate. These plans were organized as not-for-profit entities and were therefore exempt from taxes. Although originally suspicious and antagonistic toward the concept of health insurance, physicians soon came to realize that health insurance was likely to be an important factor in the payment of medical bills. By the early 1940s groups of physicians working with Blue Cross organizations had developed "Blue Shield" plans that covered certain physician fees for services provided to patients while in the hospital. Eventually most physician services, both inpatient and outpatient, came to be covered by Blue Shield and other physician coverage insurance plans.

As more and more health insurance plans developed, including those from commercial insurers, the health insurance industry soon became the "third-party payer" that exerted increasing influence over fees and prices, as well as exerting significant influence over patterns of usage within the system. The importance of the health insurance companies was greatly enhanced during the 1950s and later when generous tax reforms allowed large industries to offer health insurance as a benefit that was tax exempt to the industry and to the recipients. Employers found in health insurance plans a way to exercise their responsibility for their workers' well-being which could serve as a surrogate or substitute for wage increases. For this reason union negotiations with a number of important industries have often included healthcare benefits as an important (and occasionally the only) aspect to be considered in a new contract.

Not only employers, but the government as well, recognized the growing importance of the HCO as a contributor to the social weal. Employers were offering health benefits to the employed; but how could the society equalize access to medical care to its unemployed citizens, medical care heavily localized in the HCO? One attempt to answer this question was the rapid increase in attention of the federal government. In 1946, Congress passed the Hill-Burton Act, which encouraged the building and equipping of local community hospitals by subsidizing these endeavors. The Hill-Burton Act expired in 1978, but by that time it had stimulated the building of 500,000 hospital beds, many of which were in small and medium-sized communities. Not only community health, but also medical research was centered in the HCO, and as a mechanism for wider support to the burgeoning medical enterprise, the National Institutes of Health grew enormously following the Second World War. Since the mid-1960s there has been an ever increasing attention to federally sponsored medical research, thereby increasing the influence of the federal government on health care generally and upon those HCOs involved in medical research particularly.*

However, it was not until 1965, when the initial Medicare and Medicaid bills were passed, that the federal government became directly involved in the financing of health care for individuals. Medicare, which was initially conceived as a limited health insurance for the elderly, expanded during the legislative process into a more comprehensive package of benefits for a range of otherwise uninsured populations, including payment of major portions of the costs of hospitalization and physicians' fees. To ensure the passage of Medicare against strong opposition, determination of appropriate costs of hospitalization was based on a per diem cost per patient, with the authority for the hospital to add appropriate marginal costs; and both Medicare and Medicaid were structured to accommodate organized medicine with a fee-for-service payment mechanism. The administration of Medicare, including paying and auditing hospitals and physicians, was relegated to a particular insurance company in a specific geographic area. The choice of the insurance company that would be selected to fulfill this administrative work was left chiefly to the physicians and hospitals in that area.

---

*The mission of the National Institutes of Health is to uncover new knowledge that will lead to better health for everyone. NIH works toward that mission by: conducting research in its own laboratories; supporting the research of nonfederal scientists in universities, medical schools, hospitals, and research institutions throughout the country and abroad; helping in the training of research investigators; and fostering communication of biomedical information.

The NIH is one of eight health agencies of the Public Health Service which, in turn, is part of the U.S. Department of Health and Human Services. Comprised of twenty-four separate institutes, centers, and divisions, NIH has seventy-five buildings on more than three hundred acres in Bethesda, Maryland. From a total of about $300 in 1887, the NIH budget has grown to more than $13.6 billion in 1998. For more information visit the NIH Web pages at *http://www.nih.gov/*.

Medicaid mandated health insurance for those on welfare and for the medically indigent. The federal government and the states shared costs of this program, with the states maintaining most of the authority to set the specific benefit package offered and to set payment amounts for hospital care and physicians' fees. Medicare and Medicaid have afforded a number of positive benefits for the elderly and poor. However the adoption of a cost-based, fee-for-service reimbursement system for these programs stimulated increasing use of the healthcare system with a concomitant ballooning of costs. National health expenditures rose from $26.9 billion to $73.2 billion from 1960 to 1970. Per capita healthcare spending rose from 141 dollars to 341 dollars. Of the 1960 per capita amount, the federal government paid 15 dollars, or about 10 percent. In 1970 the federal government's share had risen to 83 dollars, or about 25 percent (HCFA statistics, 1997).

It was inevitable that after the institution of Medicare and Medicaid in 1965 the government would become a major player in the economics of health care. This involvement subsequently took two pathways: major expenditures to make the benefits of modern health care more widely accessible, and repeated, usually unsuccessful, attempts at reform of healthcare delivery in an effort to reduce the rapidly increasing costs. Federal spending increased not only because of the enactment of Medicare and Medicaid, but also because of federally subsidized building of hospitals under the Hill-Burton Act, favorable tax treatment of employer investments in health insurance benefits, NIH funding, and attractive loans and grants to medical schools and others designed to expand the supply of physicians.

During this period various U.S. presidents attempted to introduce measures to control and redistribute costs. Dwight D. Eisenhower, while vested in the success of the private, voluntary healthcare insurance system, understood its limitations with respect to the poor and the elderly who could not pay the required premiums. His proposals for government assistance to the poor and elderly were met with indifference and even outrage by some citizens and their congressional representatives. However, two federal health insurance programs were passed into law during Eisenhower's presidency. The first provided government health insurance to military dependents. The key to its success, however, was its commitment to use the Blues as administrators of the program so that the traditional fee-for-service system was not disrupted. The second piece of legislation was the Federal Employees Health Benefit Program (FEHBP) which offered federal workers a choice among multiple health insurance plans (Simmons, 1992, p. 183).

In 1968, Lyndon Johnson requested that Congress correct what he called the major deficiencies of the healthcare system, which he believed encouraged hospitalization, perpetuated the fee-for-service physician payment system, and engaged in the practice of reimbursing hospitals on the basis of costs (Simmons, 1992, p. 288). Congress declined to act on Johnson's request.

In 1969, a newly elected President Richard Nixon declared a "massive crisis" in health care. Following this declaration a debate was initiated, and the perspectives of major payers for health care (government and employers), recipients of health care (patients), and providers of health care (physicians and hospitals) were crystallized. The issue of cost containment became a major concern for each of these groups. Increasingly, major payers demanded more accountability from insurers who were the primary administrators of healthcare system payments. Up to this point insurers had maintained a passive role in the delivery of health care, and now were suddenly expected to "manage" the system in a cost-effective way. Patient recipients and providers of healthcare services had markedly different perspectives from payers for healthcare services. They advocated for increased access and quality (technology) with cost as no object. Special-interest groups representing each perspective became entrenched forces affecting the structure and delivery of health care.

The average American citizen, who had for the most part been protected from increases in the costs of health care through employer-sponsored insurance plans, remained unaware of the differing perspectives concerning cost, access, and quality of health care and how these differing perspectives added to the complexity of the healthcare system.

Nixon was a believer in the efficiency of American business, so it was natural that he sought to base healthcare reform within a market concept rather than to try to align the agendas of the different interest groups. In 1973, with Nixon's strong support, the HMO Act was passed. We will discuss its implications in the next section.

Development of managed care

There have been attempts throughout the century to establish models for physician and hospital reimbursement other than the fee-for-service model endorsed by professional societies and adopted by the Blue Cross/Blue Shield and commercial insurance plans. Increasing costs and the fear of increasing costs were the primary considerations leading to these attempts. By the mid-1920s, business, civic, and government leaders understood that the loss of income from illness combined with the relatively high costs of medical care posed a real threat to the stability of low- and middle-class families (Greenlick et al., 1988). Further, the culture was changing as more people moved to the cities from rural America. As these cultural changes accelerated, leaders began to understand that access to medical care could be a problem for larger numbers of families.

In 1926 eight prestigious foundations funded grants totaling a million dollars to form the Committee on the Cost of Medical Care (CCMC), which was to study the system of health care and to make recommendations for financing reform. Recipients of these grants included leaders in medicine, public health, and the social sciences. In 1932 the CCMC released its final report, which included recommendations that the government have a role in the planning, coordination, and delivery of health care, and that a form of either insurance or taxation be initiated for the payment of health care. At various times since the CCMC report, government leaders have made similar recommendations.

Special-interest groups, such as the American Medical Association, which as an organization has been quite successful in shaping the HCO to its interests, were antagonistic toward these recommendations and were a significant force in blocking their implementation. Without question, AMA leaders saw any sort of government role in the practice, development, or coordination of medical delivery as a threat to physician and patient autonomy; as a threat to the "right" of a patient to select his or her physician; as a threat to the "right" of the physician to accept the patient into his practice; as a threat to the physician's ability to treat the patient without governmental interference; and in particular, as a threat to the "right" of the physician to set his own fees.

By 1926, the AMA was highly organized and it controlled, with varying degrees of effectiveness, the licensing, education, and training of physicians in the whole country. The major mechanism of control exercised by the AMA was through local medical societies and their requirements for membership. Membership in local medical societies was generally necessary in order for a physician to obtain medical malpractice insurance. Thus, expulsion or membership denial from the local medical society essentially put an end to a physician's career. These local societies were often linked to the AMA and required that a local society member also be a member of the AMA.

Since as we have seen the HCO was heavily dominated by physician values throughout this period, the adoption of the "medical staff" model of hospital governance aligned the HCOs with the physicians, so the American Hospital Association joined the AMA in its opposition to any prepaid healthcare plans other than Blue Cross and Blue Shield or commercial insurance (Shadid, 1956). The AMA's stance on payment mechanisms other than fee-for-service had been decreed in 1912 when it declared as unethical "an agreement between a physician or group of physicians, as principals or agents, and a corporation, organization . . . or individual, to furnish . . . medical services to a group or class of individuals on the basis of a fee schedule, or for a salary or a fixed rate per capita" (F. Goldman, 1948, p. 59). The AMA was to prove a persistent opponent of any sort of government effort at healthcare reform that affected these areas.*

---

*In 1954, at the annual meeting of the AMA, a motion to affirm the unrestricted freedom of a patient to choose his own physician was passed, and the AMA appointed a special Commission on Medical Care Plans to be chaired by Dr. Leonard Larson. Larson and his commission undertook an exhaustive four-year study that focused on an inquiry into three issues:

1. the nature and methods of operation of the various types of plans through which persons received the services of physicians;
2. the effect of those plans on the quality and quantity of medical care provided; and

Although the CCMC failed to offer a model that could immediately be implemented, several pioneer health maintenance organizations (HMOs) were formed between 1920 and the early 1940s. The most recognized examples of these early HMOs are the Community Hospital Association of Elk City, Oklahoma, founded by Dr. Michael Shadid with the cooperation of the Farmers' Union in Beckham County; the Group Health Association (GHA) of Washington, D.C.: and the Kaiser Permanente programs that originated in Oregon, Washington, and California. The Elk City plan was formed as a cooperative; the Kaiser programs were initially formed to attend to the medical needs of groups of Kaiser employees, although it later offered general enrollment to the public; and the Group Health Association had its roots in government-sponsored healthcare reform. Even though these three plans differed ideologically, all three relied on the concept of prepaid group practices.

By the mid-1940s it was clear that these early prepayment plans would survive in spite of the opposition of organized medicine. Dr. Shadid and his physician associates, with the political support of the governor of Oklahoma, "Alfalfa Bill" Murray, and the farmers' union, were able to withstand the threat of expulsion from their local medical society. Group Health Association, initiated by I.S. Falk, who had served on the CCMC, and who had joined the new Social Security Administration under Roosevelt, obtained help from the U.S. Justice Department's Anti-Trust Division when that plan's only surgeon was expelled from the Washington, D.C. medical society. Evidence collected by the Anti-Trust Division with the help of GHA resulted in a successful suit against the AMA and the District of Columbia Medical Society, who were found guilty of violating the Sherman Anti-Trust Act.

Dr. Garfield had joined with Henry Kaiser during World War II to organize the delivery of health care to the new Kaiser shipyards. The HMO structure of prepaid fees and employed salaried healthcare professionals that Garfield developed served over 200,000 workers and their dependents during this period. At war's end, both Garfield and Kaiser were committed to continuing the program, which they saw as a model of healthcare reform. In 1945, the program was renamed the

---

3. the legal and ethical status of the arrangements used by the various plans. (Simmons, 1992, p. 177)

The commission examined the performance of Blue Cross and Blue Shield programs, indemnity programs, industry programs, student health services, and prepaid group practices. In 1959, it released its report. The report found that the quality of medical care provided within the scope of benefits offered by prepaid plans was good. It further acknowledged that the traditional freedom of the patient to choose his own physician *also* included the right of a patient to choose a system of medical care or a particular prepaid plan. The report was significant in that the AMA acknowledged formally that differing forms of delivery of healthcare services would and could compete in the provider market, and that the traditional delivery of healthcare services through fee-for-service was in some instances being abused.

Kaiser Permanente Medical Care Program, and enrollment was offered to the general public, not just employees of Kaiser Industries. In 1947 the California Medical Board temporarily suspended Dr. Garfield's license, and various other Permanente physicians were denied membership in their local medical societies. Public reaction and strong support by the labor movement helped Permanente to survive the attacks.

By 1960 independent HMOs had established their legal right to compete in the healthcare market and had attracted over 3 million subscribers, or just over 5 percent of the total insured population (Simmons, 1992, p. 130). These early managed care organization models demonstrated their efficiency in controlling costs. Kaiser Permanente Medical Care hospital utilization rates were less than 50 percent of the Blue Cross and indemnity insurance utilization rates (p. 157). The HMO plans were attractive to labor because they offered relatively comprehensive benefits, an emphasis on prevention, and utilized "community rating" extensively*
(p. 159).

Despite their demonstrated success at cost containment, the early HMOs remained a minority movement, considered by some as a utopian ideal and by other segments of the population as the first step on the road to socialized medicine.

As the costs of health care increased dramatically following World War II, two key themes repeatedly surfaced. First, in spite of increasing calls for accountability from various states, the Blues were structurally unable to challenge increases in physician and hospital costs. Second, the Blues and commercial insurers could not subsidize high-risk populations and remain competitive. By 1960, it was evident that some groups, primarily the elderly and the poor, would remain less than fully covered by the system of voluntary insurance.

Various governmental reforms were suggested, several of which were discussed in the previous section. It was Nixon who succeeded in providing some legislative support for HMOs through passage in 1973 of the HMO Act, an attempt to base healthcare reform within a market concept rather than try to accommodate the agendas of special-interest groups. The HMO Act encouraged the formation of market-based HMOs, and promised support through grants and low-interest loans. But, under this law, certification by the Office of Health Maintenance Organizations would be required in order to obtain the promised funding. Specific conditions for certification were open enrollment, community rating, comprehensive benefits, and consumer board participation. None of the nation's premier prototype HMO programs sought certification, believing that agreement to these

*Community rating refers to the idea that all members within some defined community should pay the same price for healthcare services regardless of age or preexisting conditions. The Blues were founded on this principle and so were at a competitive disadvantage with commercial insurance, who relied on the concept of experience rating, which sets payment depending on the individual's healthcare history. Thus, commercial insurers were able to offer much lower rates to more attractive populations.

conditions could result in bankruptcy (Simmons, 1992, p. 352). Nevertheless, the HMO Act did signal to organized medicine that serious reform was on its way.

The period from 1970 to 1980 was characterized by market-based reforms based on competition and reinforced by state and federal initiatives. Reformers looked to the market to control costs. Except for the continuing efforts of a few prominent politicians to keep it alive as an option, universal coverage was dropped from the nation's agenda.

But a spiral of increasing costs was financially devastating many of the Blues. Their dual role in serving provider interests while simultaneously providing a fair service to their members at a reasonable price was increasingly under question both philosophically and practically. As the numbers of Blues decreased, they sought to separate, and were eventually successful in separating, their interests from provider interests. Many Blues themselves initiated HMO programs as an alternative to their traditional fee-for-service indemnity programs. Numerous commercial insurers entered the field and the number of HMOs increased from 75 HMO-like entities in 1973 to 236 HMOs in 1980 with a total on the latter date of 9.1 million subscribers.

Managed care organizations are defined by law as insurance organizations, which is how they are listed in the Standard Industrial Classification System maintained by the Occupation Safety and Health Administration of the Department of Labor:

> 6324 Hospital and Medical Service Plans
>
> Establishments primarily engaged in providing hospital, medical and other health services to subscribers or members in accordance with prearranged agreements or service plans. Generally, these service plans provide benefits to subscribers or members in return for specified subscription charges. The plans may be through a contract under which a participating hospital or physician agrees to render the covered services without charging any additional fees. Other plans provide for partial indemnity and service benefits. Also included in this industry are separate establishments of health maintenance organizations which provide medical insurance. (*http://www.osha.gov/cgi-bin/sic/sicer?6324*)

As insurance companies MCOs are, through the 1948 McCurran-Ferguson Act, exempt from the Sherman Act, the Clayton Act, the Federal Trade Commission Act (15 U.S.C. 41 et seq.), and the Act of June 19, 1936, known as the Robinson-Patman Anti-Discrimination Act. Thus, except for any agreement to boycott, coerce, or intimidate, or any act of boycott, coercion, or intimidation, MCOs are exempt from federal antitrust law. In contrast, HCOs are not exempt from antitrust law, and the decade from 1970 to 1980 saw competition (cost containment) promoted by the federal government through various challenges to healthcare providers (primarily HCOs) based on antitrust concepts.

The two major purchasers of healthcare services, the government and large employers, had by the period from 1980 to 1993 succeeded in differentiating their interests from the interests of organized medicine. The payment of hospital and other institutional providers at their per diem "cost" was early on identified as a primary cause of healthcare cost inflation. To control the huge growth in Medicare and Medicaid, the Health Care Financing Administration (HFCA) changed its system for reimbursing hospitals from per diem cost to a "prospective payment system" (PPS) in 1983. Under PPS, hospitals received a fixed payment for each patient treated using diagnosis-related groupings (DRGs) to determine the payment amount (Simmons, 1992, p. 401). The theory behind the PPS system parallels the theory that governs "capitation." It was expected that PPS would provide an incentive for hospitals to manage themselves more effectively. Under this system hospitals were free to keep any payment surplus but were forced to make up the difference if the actual cost of the service rendered was greater than the amount allowed by HFCA. The result was dramatic. Length of stay for Medicare patients dropped from 10 days in 1983 to 8.5 days in 1989 and all indications were that the quality of care received by Medicare patients was good in spite of this decrease in length of stay (p. 402).

But hospitals, in addition to becoming more efficient, increasingly turned to the practice of "cost shifting" through the 1980s. Hospitals shifted their shortfall in costs of caring for government-sponsored patients to private insurers who were required to pay more than the Medicare patients. This practice may partially explain why American business views proposals for universal coverage with such suspicion since they fear they will bear the brunt of the costs (Simmons, 1992, p. 405).

Government bureaucrats in control of healthcare payments began to adjust DRG payments so that they did not keep up with increases in hospital costs. By 1991 more than half of U.S. HCOs were losing money on Medicare patients. Wishing to achieve the same savings with physician fees that the imposition of PPS had achieved with hospital fees, in 1989 Congress approved a new payment system for physicians other than the previously established "usual and customary" fee plan. This new payment system, the "resource-based relative-value scale" (RBRVS), along with the PPS system gave HFCA the ability to set fees for government-sponsored patients for both physicians and hospitals.

The private sector was also changing. Although the government enjoyed some temporary success in controlling the growth rate of costs in Medicare and Medicaid in the 1980s, this was not the case for American businesses. In 1965 corporate America was paying roughly $8.40 per $100 of pretax profit for healthcare benefits for its workers. By late 1989, that figure had risen to $56.40 per hundred dollars of pretax profit (Lipson, 1993).

One avenue for cost savings by large companies was to take advantage of the 1974 Employee Retirement Income Security Act (ERISA), which exempts those employers who "self-insure" their health benefit plans from state regulation, taxation, and control. Under these self-insured plans, the employer pays the healthcare claims directly, rather than purchasing an insurance policy to pay claims, thus escaping dependence on state-regulated insurance companies, which are often more expensive. (http://www.managedcaremag.com/archiveMC/9705/9795.erisa.shtml). These companies either formed or turned to MCOs to manage their plans.

All of the aforementioned factors were in place when the Clinton plan failed to pass Congress in 1994, leaving only "the market" to address the economic and social issues surrounding the healthcare system. Since then the growth of managed care plans has been staggering. Estimates vary, but it is generally conceded that since 1990 the average annual national growth rate of managed care enrollment exceeds 16 percent (Virginia Health Maintenance Organizations Directory, 1997, p. 6). This has been at the expense of traditional indemnity insurance, which has sharply declined from more than 50 percent of numbers insured in 1993 to less than 30 percent in 1995 (ibid.). Roughly 75 percent of American workers are currently enrolled in some form of managed care plan. Managed care provides services to roughly 40 percent of Medicaid beneficiaries and Medicare has about 13 percent of beneficiaries in managed care plans (Colby, 1997). There is evidence that managed care to date has been able to slow the rate of growth of healthcare costs, but questions remain over whether this decreased rate of growth can continue without materially downgrading the quality of healthcare services.

Ethical climate in the postwar HCO

As we noted in the preceding sections, influence on the external and internal ethical climate of HCOs is not independent of the source of the financial support for those institutions. When the major support of hospitals was from their community or religious sponsors, the mediators of their values to the institution, usually a board of trustees determined the values for the institution. As hospitals developed closer relationships with physicians and their services began to constitute a major source of income for the institutions, the values and mission of those hospitals became more closely identified with the professional values of the clinicians who were central to their function.

Although we have not emphasized this aspect of hospital development, it is very clear that by the beginning of our postwar period, hospitals were the locus of an extremely expensive (and very profitable) intersection of industries: the pharmaceutical industry, the medical technology industry, and several service industries as well—all at the service of physicians and their patients. The intimacy of the relation of medical practice and medical facilities was a double-edged partnership; the hospitals needed the doctors, and the doctors needed the hospitals. It was an increasingly expensive partnership as well; and many of the questions that began to dominate in this period circled around a very important issue: how will medical care be financed?

As government required a complicated set of administrative, financial, and auditing procedures; as attention to patient rights required constant attention to these issues; as increasingly costly technology and operation in a competitive environment became paramount for continued operation; and as physicians became more specialized and less able and interested in the operational aspects of the HCO, administrative personnel were required to increase their attention to and their influence in the overall direction and day-to-day operation of the HCO as well as the hospital's status in the community. This meant that administrators with varying amounts of input from trustees, medical staffs, and others (nurses, attorneys, others from within and beyond the HCO) began to have more and more power within the institution—a trend which by the end of this period began to give them a dominant role in shaping the HCO's ethical climate. As physicians became increasingly specialized they had less possibility for independence from the hospital, which was the repository of and mediator for all the increasingly expensive tools of medical specialization, as well as of medical education and research.

Most mission statements, the stated bases for the internal ethical climate, continued to pay homage to the traditional goals and activities expected of hospitals, and now the growing cadre of professional administrators committed themselves to those values. From the first stage of hospital development in the United States, the value of providing some degree of medical treatment even to the poorest of citizens survived in goals such as "care for the patient without regard to ability to pay," and from the second stage, identification of hospital values with professional values encouraged such claims as "each patient is our area for attention and we are committed to giving each patient the best care possible." But hospitals confronted increasing dissonance in allowing all clinical decisions to be made without reference to business issues; in spite of these high-sounding phrases, during times of financial stress HCOs reverted to a business perspective and became more concerned about fiscal survival than about particular interventions for specific patients.

Although clinical treatment was becoming increasingly dependent upon the growing influence of the HCO, the postwar HCO was still very much dominated by the values of the earlier period, given priority by the increasingly powerful administrators, as well as by the clinical professionals. By now the population to whom the HCO was expected to deliver "the best care possible" was the whole society, not just the wealthy, and employers and government contributed to the growing expense of doing so. That the expense eventually grew faster than the willingness was in large part because of the virtues and successes of the medical enterprise. People associated with the healthcare industry felt they were doing something valuable which was appreciated by their society, and many people think of the postwar period as the "golden age" of medicine. We were told to heal and, to cure, and we did; to be suddenly told, as we were at the end of this period, "But we didn't mean for you to do it *that* successfully" (or, more particularly, "that expensively") was, not surprisingly, viewed as an inconsistency.

The 1980s and early 1990s have seen increased governmental attention and influence leading to more bureaucratic attempts to satisfy governmental and accrediting agencies. The previous attachment of the HCO to its community became less important and less obvious. The pressures of increasing healthcare costs in the 1980s and early 1990s forced attention to the bottom line at all levels of operation of every HCO, including the clinical level. The business dimensions of health care became paramount issues, and how patient care issues and professional issues were to be addressed within this context was an open question; a question that the Clinton administration attempted to answer in 1993 with its ill-fated attempt to institute a complicated "managed care competition" plan of national scope. There was little in this plan to enhance the ethical climate of HCOs, and its concentration on access and cost-saving issues without allowing for traditional values to operate within healthcare organizations likely contributed to its demise.

By the time Clinton acknowledged that his vision of healthcare reform would fail, the healthcare system was in ethical disarray. What it should and did stand for, how these values were to be inculcated within organizations and reinforced by daily activities, were not only a puzzle to the industry as a whole, but they were of less than passing interest to many in positions of power in individual HCOs. Survival in the new era was the most compelling issue. The traditional hospital, nursing home, and doctor of previous times were considered anachronisms that had little to offer in modern healthcare management. It was, and in our view remains, a time of crisis without an accepted source of moral guidance for the HCO, for those who go there for medical help, and for those who work there. The shift to managed care in the private sector of the economy is, by default, an attempt toward solving these problems. There have also been efforts by governmental regulators, accrediting agencies such as the JCAHO and the AHA to foster positive changes in the operation of HCOs. Despite the potential of these institutions outside of the HCO to encourage beneficial and stabilizing changes, we believe that each HCO must actively address the many problems facing the modern healthcare system and develop internal mechanisms of organization ethics.

7

The Ethical Climate in Today's Healthcare Organization

Health care and the issues surrounding its delivery have been a source of recurring concern for the American people. Americans ranked healthcare reform in 1992 polls right after the economy and foreign affairs as an issue that should be addressed by presidential candidates (Skocpol, 1995, p. 68). Not surprisingly, Bill Clinton, in his presidential campaign that year, promised to put this issue high on his agenda. In September 1993, during the first year of his presidency, Clinton called on both Congress and the American people to fix a broken healthcare system—to give every American health security that "is always there, health care that can never be taken away" (p. 67).

During the next few months the president, his wife Hillary Rodham Clinton, and a number of recognized health system experts tried to develop a plan to address the systemic problems of healthcare delivery. The two major issues were increasing costs and reduced access, so Clinton looked for a way to push the employer-based U.S. healthcare system toward cost-efficiency and universal coverage (Skocpol, 1995, p. 69). The task force he appointed adopted the model of "managed competition" to combine the efficiencies of managed care with regional healthcare purchasing agencies, universal access to care, and payment derived in part from tax increases. Mr. Clinton believed he had a mandate to proceed along these lines. For a number of political and social reasons he was proven to be wrong.

After the defeat of this plan in 1994, it was clear that comprehensive, government-sponsored healthcare reform would no longer be part of the national agenda, at least for the next few years. Reformers, regulators, and business interests had no real choice except to look to the market to provide a way of providing a structure of healthcare delivery that would be more cost-effective and economically predictable than the existing structure. Since some of the older managed-care organizations had already demonstrated a record of success in restraining the costs of health care, many employers turned to MCOs as an economically stable way of providing healthcare benefits for their employees. The government also endorsed this approach and is presently supporting pilot programs administered by MCOs as a way of restraining the growth of healthcare costs in Medicare, Medicaid, and military healthcare plans for the populations receiving healthcare benefits under these programs.

The death of the Clinton plan in 1994 represents for us another shift in HCO stakeholder relationships. But rather than a shift among stakeholder relationships occurring *within* the HCO as a result of a change in the values endorsed by society—power has moved *outside* the HCO to those who regulate and purchase healthcare services. This power, by and large, now resides in federal and state governments and in American businesses, the large-scale purchasers of healthcare insurance. This shift in the site and exercise of power occurred chiefly in response to the perceived need for cost-containment mechanisms, but it presumed that the fundamental values which define health care would remain unaffected. This presumption was, at least in hindsight, unrealistic. The values of an organization are influenced by the locus of power among the stakeholders of that organization. These stakeholders can be both internal and external to the organization. If the locus of power changes, values that are dependent on that power can change. The result, we believe, is an unresolved moral climate within the HCO where there is much confusion about its appropriate roles in today's healthcare landscape.

To understand the external factors that influence the internal organizational climate of today's HCO, we need to look more closely at them. In this chapter we will begin by discussing how the public currently views the healthcare system and why a vigorous public debate on how to prioritize or define important values in medical care seems unlikely. Then we will discuss more thoroughly than in the preceding chapter the contractual relationships that define MCOs. We will also outline some of the new methods of financing and management that characterize these relationships and assess the effects of these methods on both the HCO and its stakeholders, including patients. Finally, we will consider the effects of accrediting standards and how the HCO has responded to these systemic changes within the context of society's failure to define acceptable health care and the moral parameters that should guide its delivery.

HOW CITIZENS VIEW THE SYSTEM

The National Coalition on Health Care (NCHC) describes itself as "the nation's largest and most broadly representative alliance working to improve America's health care." The coalition, which was founded in 1990 and is nonprofit and rigorously nonpartisan, consists of almost one hundred groups, employing or representing approximately 100 million Americans. In a policy study, "A Reality Check: The Public's Changing View of our Health Care System," the NCHC states that a summary of twenty-two other national surveys taken between April 1996 and January 1998 reveals a clear pattern. Consumer concerns about health care are increasing and have grown from a narrow focus with individual elements of the healthcare system to broader, system-wide concerns. People are worried about:

1. Their present and future ability to pay for health insurance and medical care
2. The increasing difficulty of gaining access to necessary care when coverage is lacking or inadequate
3. The quality of medical care

In a 1997 coalition survey, thirteen statements dealt directly with perceptions of the quality of health care. The vast majority of Americans agreed with the statement "There is something seriously wrong with our healthcare system," 87 percent agreed that "the quality of medical care for the average person needs to be improved," and *only 15 percent* had "complete confidence" in hospital care. Less than half of the respondents said they had "confidence in the health care system to take care of me." (Access http://www.nchc.org for an executive summary of the report.)

Although many Americans are worried about the current healthcare system and the HCO, most insured people are satisfied with their own healthcare plans (Blendon et al., 1998, p. 83). While a number of explanations have been offered for this apparent inconsistency we believe that these surveys demonstrate the conflicting or unresolved values Americans have concerning health care and the system that supports it. Increases in the cost of medical care have heightened the underlying tension between ideas of liberty and equality. On the one hand, a libertarian perspective suggests that health care is a commodity like any other and should be bought and sold in an open market. On the other, a more egalitarian perspective holds that health care represents a different kind of good—a good that should be shared as equally as possible. Trying to satisfactorily address these issues means considering justice and allocation issues in healthcare delivery. It means rethinking the basic premise of entitlement in health care. It means deciding on and prioritizing the values we think are important in medical care. Unfortunately, the schism that exists between the public's view of the healthcare system and the individual's satisfaction with its delivery means that looking to the general public for help in clarifying fundamental values upon which to base an ethical climate in an HCO is likely to be of little help. Education of the public as to the real questions that face all aspects of the healthcare system should help in clarifying the public's values, but it is likely that an organization ethics program in tomorrow's HCO will be the sponsor of such education rather than its beneficiary.

DEFINING THE MCO

In the last chapter we discussed the development of managed care in the twentieth century. We discussed the legal definition of managed care organizations and the laws that govern its operations. In this chapter we look more closely at the contractual relationships it forms and the implications of those relationships.

Managed care organizations (MCOs) are a broad and constantly changing array of health plans which attempt to control the cost and improve the quality of health care by coordinating medical and other health related services. Managed care is a generic term that includes health maintenance organizations (HMOs) as a type of MCO. Both MCOs and HMOs may define themselves as a "health care delivery system that accepts responsibility and financial risk for providing a specified set of services to an enrolled membership in exchange for a fixed, prepaid fee from the purchaser" (Virginia Health Maintenance Organizations Directory, 1997, p. 6).

The stated goal of MCOs is to slow the increase in costs of health care, while attempting to enhance the quality of, and in some cases the access to, the services for which it is responsible. MCOs provide an agreed-upon set of services for an agreed upon fee to a specific, contractually defined, group of subscribers. A party with responsibility for the healthcare needs of these subscribers (an employer, a government agency, or some other agency, henceforth called "payer") pays this fee, or at least a major portion of it, to the MCO. Certain standards of quality are generally promised in the delivered services, and most MCOs have developed mechanisms for updating quality standards, based either on their own experience or the experience of others in the healthcare field.*

Most businesses, not directly associated with health care can easily identify a single group as the consumer of their product or service. This allows companies to develop very specific profiles of that customer group as a first step in under-

---

*Most MCOs are accredited by the National Committee for Quality Assurance (NCQA). One requirement for accreditation is that members have mechanisms in place to report on the quality of care delivered.

standing the quality needs of the customer. But MCOs try to meet the needs and expectations of two sets of customers:

1. Payers: the entity with which the MCO has contracted, often an employer or agency
2. Recipients of care: the individuals within the subscriber group who actually receive the healthcare benefits; actual and potential patients

These two groups have different concerns and so can be expected to assign different priorities to the objectives of the MCO. Generally the payer will be more concerned with the total cost of providing healthcare benefits to the group for which it is responsible. The payer will be concerned with the *number* of people served and the *cost* of the services delivered to that group. The actual or potential patient will be more concerned by the *quality* and *quantity* of the services delivered by the MCO. Quality issues for many patients include choice of provider, freedom to change providers, and access to the best available treatment modalities (regardless of cost).

The MCO operates on the assumption that there is no inherent contradiction in trying to meet the expectations of these two different sets of customers. The argument they make is that the quality needs of the subscriber group can be met while at the same time meeting the cost needs of the payer. This argument is based on a philosophy of business that was made popular by W. Deming called "total quality management" (TQM). (See Chapter 10 for a fuller discussion of TQM.) This concept serves as the philosophical basis for the aforementioned claim made by MCOs and is used to buttress the argument that health care can be better managed than in the past. Advocates argue that by focusing on the processes by which a good or service is produced beginning at the "source" of the production stream, cost savings can be made while simultaneously improving the quality of the product or service. MCOs argue that this approach allows them to satisfy the cost objectives of the payer of healthcare services while satisfying the quality needs of the actual or potential patient.

Other major stakeholders directly affected by the activities of a MCO are the healthcare providers (either individual healthcare professionals or HCOs) who contractually agree to deliver to the patient group the healthcare services contracted for by the employer or government agency. Even though contractual relationships will vary, the individuals or organizations delivering these healthcare services can be considered, in business terms, suppliers to the MCO. It is important to note that the greater the volume of income derived by the supplier from one source, the more vulnerable that supplier is in a contractual relationship with that source. Therefore healthcare providers who rely on a single MCO contract for a large portion of their income are very susceptible to economic coercion from the MCO.

Several different contractual relationships between professional providers and MCOs have become common: group model HMOs, staff model HMOs, and IPA model HMOs. They are defined below.

- Group model HMOs contract with independent groups of physicians or other providers to provide coordinated care for large numbers of HMO patients for a fixed, per-member fee. These groups will often care for the members of several HMOs. Group model HMOs refer to a *network* of physicians that may include IPAs *(see below)*.

- Staff model HMO employ salaried physicians and other health professionals who provide care solely for members of one HMO, and who are the primary (often the only) source of care for these subscribers. Many early HMOs were staff model HMOs.

- Independent Practice Associations (IPA) are groups of independent physicians who work in their own offices. These independent practitioners provide a full range of services for HMO members and are compensated via a per-member payment (called "capitation") from the HMO or deliver services to the HMO's patients based on some type of discounting arrangement. These providers often care for members of many HMOs, as well as for patients with other types of payment mechanisms.

A growing number of HMOs now offer a point-of-service (POS) option in addition to one or more of the above payment methods. These "escape hatch" plans allow HMO members to seek care from physicians not affiliated with the HMO, thus satisfying patient preferences for choice of physician; but the premiums for POS plans are much more costly than those for HMO plans that restrict the choice of physician. Moreover, when an HMO member receives care from a nonparticipating physician or hospital, the HMO normally pays far less than 100 percent coverage of necessary medical services (i.e., the patient is responsible for a portion of the charge) (http://www.wnet.org/archive/mhc/Info/Glossary/Glossary.html#HMP).

The gross income of the MCO (HMO) is the difference between the amount of money it receives for the delivery of health care and the actual cost of delivering that care. MCOs relieve the payer from assuming the financial risk of providing a certain set of services to a defined population. "Risk" means the possibility that the subscriber pool may incur more medical expenses than has been foreseen for that group. The advantage to the payer is that, at least in the short term, the payer knows exactly the cost of providing healthcare benefits. Since MCOs operate financially on the difference between the fee it receives for the promise of delivery of healthcare services and the actual cost of delivery, they have a powerful incentive to control the costs of healthcare delivery.

MCOs seek to control the costs of delivering healthcare services to the subscriber group both by controlling expenditures directly related to providing these services and by seeking to limit unnecessary medical costs associated with a subscriber group. Controlling expenditures directly related to provided healthcare services can occur through such efficient business practices as volume buying or insistence on discounts for provider services. It can occur through the application of business management techniques like TQM to healthcare administration and through attempts of the MCO to increase (or limit) the numbers of its subscriber pool.

Controlling costs by seeking to limit unnecessary medical care can occur through reliance on provider protocols or by the implementation of such ideas as case management. It can occur through attempts to manage demand for healthcare services, for instance, by requiring relatively high copayments from the subscriber patient. The MCO can also seek to control what it deems to be unnecessary medical care by shifting or sharing the risk of higher than anticipated costs with something or someone other than itself. One method of risk shifting or risk sharing is attempting to alter or influence provider behavior. The more ethically problematic of these techniques are discussed in greater detail below.

NEW METHODS OF FINANCING AND MANAGING HEALTH CARE

Before 1994 many Americans had never heard of managed care or health maintenance organizations. This rapidly changed as new MCOs were formed to compete in the market-based healthcare economy after the failure of the Clinton plan. Many of these new MCOs approached the market aggressively. In spite of an often critical press and a confused public, these MCOs touted their ability to provide efficient, reasonably priced health care. But few attempts were made to enlighten the general public about the mechanisms used by MCOs in the delivery of cost-efficient care: mechanisms such as constraints on provider disclosure and devices that seek to influence provider behavior.

An example of a constraint on provider disclosure are the so-called gag clauses, which prevent the provider from discussing with patients treatment plans that are not covered by the plan, or prevent the provider from discussing with patients financial incentives which could affect the patient's care (Council Report, 1995). Gag clauses and their potential impact on patient care have received much attention by the press and, as a result, legislation concerning gag clauses is being debated in Congress and anti-gag-clause laws have been passed or are pending in most states. Much more troublesome to observers of the healthcare industry are devices used to influence provider behavior through various reimbursement schemes.

Types of reimbursement schemes that can be used to influence provider behavior include withholds, capitation arrangements, bonuses, and gatekeeper functions. Withholds are defined as the withholding of a certain percentage of each provider's nominal income, which, at specified intervals, may be returned to the provider, or may be pooled and divided among all of the providers. Amounts received by providers will depend on some measure of provider performance that will be defined by the plan, and linked to the overall budget allocated to the provider(s) by the plan. Capitation agreements are defined as contracts with providers under which the provider agrees to supply all of a subscriber patient's healthcare needs for a set monthly fee, thereby placing the risk for loss of income and the incentive to avoid loss solely on the provider. Bonuses are linked to plan resource surpluses and are disbursed to particular providers based on their "productivity" (defined according to quality measurements, financial measurements, or both). These agreements can be made with entire organizations like HCOs or with individual providers. They can be made between the HCO and the MCO, or between the MCO and individual providers, or between the HCO and the individual providers associated with the HCO.

The "gatekeeper" is another example of a reimbursement mechanism designed to influence provider behavior. Essentially, it is a variation of the capitation concept. Gatekeepers are usually primary-care physicians who are responsible for the overall health care of a particular subscriber to the MCO's plan and who are, therefore, responsible for the costs of that subscriber patient's care. The gatekeeper's income is linked in some fashion—either through arrangements described above or in some other fashion—to the MCO's profitability. The gatekeeper has the responsibility to refer the subscriber patient, if needed, for specialized testing or specialized care. Specialized care is always more costly, so specialized care affects the profits of the MCO and, through some linkage, the gatekeeper's income. Inherent in this arrangement is an incentive for gatekeepers to undertreat their patient as well as an incentive for gatekeepers to perform outside their realm of expertise in attempts to limit the costs associated with referrals.

It was inevitable that as knowledge about some of these mechanisms spread, the general public began to fear that MCOs were arrogant and insensitive concerning the commodity being brokered—health care. The knowledge of how these mechanisms worked raised questions in the public's mind about provider motives and their role as patient advocates. But in spite of this worry neither the public nor our political leaders have been able to frame a coherent debate about what values should be represented in the delivery of health care and how these values should be prioritized.

Patients, healthcare professionals, HCOs, and the general public have in many cases been surprised by the frenzy of MCO and HCO activity since 1994. Competition in what was now explicitly designated as a "healthcare industry" became increasingly intense. One result of this activity was a wave of conversions and consolidations of both nonprofit and for-profit healthcare plans and HCOs (Gray, 1997). The amounts of money involved in these conversions and consolidations are staggering to the average American, who although aware of the costs of individual care, had never before considered profit to be an appropriate part of the costs to the patient. Even nonprofit HCOs that intended to maintain their status and culture as nonprofits have been forced by market pressure to adopt management styles that reflected market culture and market idiom (Kleinke, 1998).

The MCO has the power, through its contractual relationships with large employers whose subscriber populations are to a great extent "captive," to insist on the aforementioned business practices, and these activities do indeed seem to be slowing the yearly increases in healthcare costs. In 1993 healthcare costs in the United States rose 7.8 percent over 1992 expenditures. This was the lowest rate of growth since 1986 and believed to be a result of the growth of managed care (Francis, 1997).

The success MCOs experienced in restraining the rate of growth of healthcare costs was in itself an assurance that market penetration of managed care plans would increase. Estimates vary, but it is generally conceded that the average annual national growth rate since 1990 of managed care enrollment exceeds 16 percent (Virginia Health Maintenance Organizations, 1997, p. 6). Businesses with two hundred or more workers had enrolled more then 81 percent of their employees in some form of managed care by 1998 (Brodie, Brady & Altman, 1998).

The shift from traditional fee-for-service insurance plans to managed care plans has meant that modern HCOs face a formidable customer for their services. Furthermore, the HCO faces this customer from an eroded financial and political platform that impedes the HCO's ability to negotiate with the MCO. Government generosity has ended. Reimbursement policies through Medicare and Medicaid have been tightened. "Cost shifting," a longstanding practice of transferring the costs of care from the government to the private sector, is no longer the option it once was for HCOs (Goldsmith, 1998). In addition, individual providers and HCOs have been unable to form relationships that could be used to counter the bargaining strength of MCOs. The Federal Trade Commission, whose mandate is to protect free trade, made it clear that associations of individual providers or HCOs whose goal included any sort of price fixing would meet with legal action based on the antitrust laws.* HCOs have been finally forced to adjust their own business strategies to meet the challenge of a new and often hostile market. The most common strategy HCOs have adopted to meet these challenges, consolidation, is discussed in a later section of this chapter.

---

*In the mid-1970s, the FTC formed a division within the Bureau of Competition to investigate potential antitrust violations involving health care services. The Health Care Services and Products Division consists of approximately twenty-five lawyers and investigators who work exclusively on healthcare antitrust matters. Health Care Division staff also work with staff in the FTC's ten regional offices on healthcare matters. Information on FTC activities can be found in "FTC Antitrust Actions In Health Care Services" at (1999) http://www.ftc.gov/bc/atahcsvs.htm.

The implementation of these new business practices in HCOs to meet the demands of their newly critical payers has represented a major disruption in the internal ethical climate of the HCO. The internal constituencies of the HCO—its professional members, its administrators, and eventually its patients—are being subjected to different expectations; different not only from the expectations of recent decades, but different sometimes from the expectations of last month. Change has been a constant theme of health care in the United States; but seldom has change been so rapid, or so externally driven. From the standpoint of the HCO, the major change is twofold: a shift in priorities and a shift of control.

The HCO has always been expected to deliver high-quality care at reasonable cost, and society is certainly justified in expecting it to do so. If in the early part of the postwar period the emphasis in that expectation was on quality, the most recent emphasis has been on cost. The HCO is being asked to deliver the same or higher quality of care for reduced cost. Thus, the priority of the HCO has shifted from quality to cost control, which is a direct result of the control exercised over HCOs by MCOs.

To understand how this shift of control manifests itself, we will look more carefully at the effect of risk shifting or risk sharing on the HCO's primary constituent—the patient. We will note some of the problematic ethical implications for HCOs and individual providers by considering some of the mechanisms used to shift or share risk.

Risk shifting and its threat to professional integrity

As mentioned earlier in this chapter, management of "risk" is one of the mechanisms used by MCOs to reach their goals. The MCO's profit is determined by the actual costs of delivering healthcare services, and the major risk threatening that profit is that the actual costs of delivering care will be greater than anticipated and therefore exceed the amount paid for by the payers. The MCO's success, indeed its survival, depends on delivering those services at a financial point that is either less than or equal to the amount paid by businesses, government, and other groups for the agreed-upon services.

The risk involved in this arrangement can be managed in several ways. Risk can be managed globally—that is by undertaking the insurance of one specified group which has a certain risk profile, or by relying on actuarial figures or using experience rating* to determine premiums. Another way of managing risk is to shift it or share it through contractual relationships with other parties. Here we are concerned with the ethical problems that the MCO may be exposed to and may expose their contractual partners to and how these problems may affect pro-

---

Experience rating refers to systems that have been developed to measure the potential risk of healthcare expenses associated with an individual or group of individuals.

fessional providers and their patients through the mechanisms of risk shifting or risk sharing.

We devise a simple model to illustrate the point, Figure 7.1. Briefly, the MCO contracts with a "payer," the government or a large employer, to deliver a set of services for which it is paid a flat fee. For simplicity we assume that the MCO contracts with an HCO to deliver these services to the group for whom the government or large employer has assumed responsibility but this relationship can be with individual providers. The MCO seeks to shift or share the risk of larger-than-anticipated healthcare costs with the HCO through some arrangement like capitation. The HCO, in turn, will seek to share or shift the risk of larger-than-anticipated costs with something or someone other than itself. The HCO, like the MCO, has every incentive to introduce a conflict of interest in its own contractual relationships with the individual providers it contracts with. The mechanisms used to introduce this conflict of interest—capitation, bonuses, withholds, and the like—have been discussed above. But the individual provider has nowhere to shift the risk of larger-than-anticipated costs of delivery except to the patient.

The threat to professional integrity lies in the reimbursement mechanism that relies on a financial advantage of the provider to undertreat and the assumption that the provider will act on the basis of his financial self-interest rather than in the interests of the patient; that the provider *will* undertreat, thus saving the system (including the provider) money. Anticipated cost savings are therefore premised on the assumed willingness of the provider to look more carefully at the amount and costs of health care. But inherent in these arrangements is the temptation for the provider, be it an individual or an organization, to abandon its commitment to the welfare of the patients served. If there is no cost saving—if the

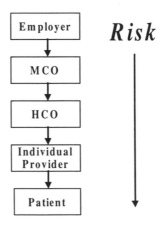

FIGURE 7.1. Structure of risk relationships.

provider, within a given interval, cannot or will not put its own welfare over that of the patient, then these risk-shifting mechanisms guarantee that actual financial disadvantage will be shared. If it is expensive to provide high-quality health care, the cost of providing that quality is shared between the provider and MCO, not just the MCO.

From the provider perspective, the outcome is a lose-lose situation. If money is saved it benefits the MCO primarily and the providers only secondarily; and the presumption of the patient and indeed the system is that the savings come because the provider has sold out. If money is not saved, the providers and the MCO share the burden of the loss. Further, a third mechanism, deselection of individual providers, allows the MCO to disencumber itself of those providers who do not contribute to the profits of the organization.

Fee-for-service medicine, it has been suggested, is the cause of our present dilemma. Fee for service provided at least a covert incentive to overtreatment. It is argued that fee for service reinforced society's unlimited demand for healthcare goods and services and hence exacerbated the costs of medical care. Whatever the truth in this argument, fee for service did have two strong moral advantages. First, it reinforced, in practice as in theory, a commitment to the value of health for its citizenry, or at least some segments of the citizenry. Second, it reinforced the basis for professional ethics in that it rewarded the individual practitioner for acting as her patients' advocate. Problems with fee for service obviously occurred when the lure of financial gain interfered with good clinical judgement and induced healthcare professionals to use treatment modalities for financial gain rather than for appropriate health care.

We spoke of conflicts of interest and conflicts of responsibility in Chapter 5, and when the provider is an individual physician, the conflict-of-interest mechanism we have just described applies. The threat to the integrity of the HCO is best understood as a conflict of commitment. The HCO is and always has been expected to deliver high-quality care for reasonable cost; the mission of the HCO, and our expectation of it, ties cost to quality. The HCO is committed to both, and decisions which affect the priority the institution gives to one or the other of those values can create a conflict of commitment in decision making. The emphasis on cost shifts the power to determine the ethical structure of the HCO to different components and stakeholders of the HCO. Unless this is explicit and open to negotiation, the commitment of the organization to the value of appropriate care can be called into question in the minds of some of the individuals both within the HCO and beyond it.

Conflicts of interest and commitment are inherent in the delivery of health care and there are no mechanisms that could adequately address all possible situations. There is one mechanism, however, which is satisfactory to most patients and providers. This is full disclosure of any conflict situation that could have an adverse effect on the care of a patient or on the professional integrity of a clinician. Full disclosure may be the only mechanism available in conflict situations. It has become the common ethical pathway for addressing these problems in the healthcare system today. Full disclosure is not always easy and may put an individual or organization in a difficult situation, but the public demands some method for oversight of the healthcare system and full disclosure is the only mechanism that is both universally available and practical.

Consolidation and its threat to institutional morale

The most significant response to the pressures for new ways of healthcare financing has been to consolidate. Consolidation can take two forms. One method is to seek affiliation with a neighboring hospital or system. This form of consolidation is commonly called a "horizontal merger." It is designed to achieve two objectives: (1) to have the clout to counter negotiations with large purchasing groups, suppliers as well as MCOs; and (2) to achieve economies of scale by spreading fixed costs over a larger number of hospital beds (Hollis, 1997).

Consolidation may also result in the vertical integration of related clinical activities, including subacute facilities, outpatient "surgicenters," rehab centers, nursing homes, assisted-living centers, and home health agencies (Kleinke, 1998). Vertical integration is attractive to third parties because of its "one-stop-shopping" appeal, as many HCOs have discovered; and it offers the potential for improved coordination of care at reduced cost. Consolidation may also involve attempts by the HCO to align physician incentives to that of the organization. One example of such an alignment occurs with equity sharing, which is the practice of giving physicians a financial stake in the organization. This provides an incentive for physician referrals to facilities in which they have equity.*

Any form of consolidation is primarily undertaken with the goal of increasing "efficiencies." This implies either an expansion of the market under consideration or the elimination of services or subfacilities that duplicate each other. In an industry characterized by excess capacity, higher productivity in the HCO is being defined by declining admissions and shorter lengths of stay. Thus, one would expect the focus of consolidation in health care, as in banks or grocery stores, to be on the elimination of duplicate services or excess capacity. This means staff reductions or reassignments.

Vertical or horizontal integration of HCOs can result in more effective utilization of available facilities, as when through consolidation with community providers a HCO can reduce the use of expensive emergency rooms for services that can be delivered more cheaply at other sites. Consolidation can improve healthcare

---

*This practice of equity sharing is explicitly addressed in the JCAHO standards. The JCAHO requires disclosure in instances where the physician refers a patient to a facility in which a financial interest is involved (Joint Commission for Accreditation of Healthcare Organizations, 1996, pp. 95–97).

delivery, as well as reduce costs; quality and cost of care need not be inversely related. However, HCO stakeholders, including patients, physicians, nurses, management, and the community, have experienced and will continue to experience the stress that accompanies change. This will be true irrespective of whether the organization handles staff reductions or reassignments brutally or in a sensitive and open fashion.

The board of trustees of the HCO involved in consolidation is under stress also and is often unable to support the stated mission and ethical climate of the HCO. During consolidation, the board may be split or be replaced entirely, with the resultant loss of continuity of leadership. Community ties based on trust, formed at the board level and forged over a period of time, may be lost as persons from outside the community replace board members. New board members will almost certainly have goals that differ from the previous board and an allegiance to the organization which has appointed them.

But even if replacement board members have the same goals as the original board, providing leadership during periods of consolidation may not be easy. For instance, if consolidation takes place between two HCOs that have spent many years competing with each other, they are not going to put aside this "historical baggage" easily and merge into a joint culture smoothly (Hollis, 1997, p. 135). Jealousies and resistance are inevitable among stakeholder groups, especially when decisions must be made as to where clinical services should be consolidated. Job security of individuals, as well as the prestige, authority, and identity of both individuals and organizations, is threatened during these periods of consolidations.

One of the first steps after consolidation may be to replace the CEO with someone new who will have authority to hire and fire senior managers. Without a doubt, senior management knows that during consolidation many friends and colleagues will be replaced as economies of scale are realized. The American College of Healthcare Executives (ACHE) has expressed its concern on the volatility of employment at the senior level in a HCO. The ACHE states that CEOs and senior administrators have to be provided some protection because of the "significant personal and financial risk" a high-level administrator assumes on accepting employment in the HCO. While the ACHE does not provide recent figures, it notes that turnover rate in senior positions in HCOs in 1992 was 14.5 percent (ache.org/policy/pps2.html). Common sense dictates that figure is probably much higher now, given the amount of industry-wide consolidation since 1992.

Staff, consulting physicians, and other clinicians face the same uncertainty as other stakeholders during periods of consolidation. In addition, the physician is often asked to make an explicit commitment to the well-being of the organization, which may conflict with other obligations, particularly those related to her professional role.

Patients, just as other stakeholders, feel the effects of efficiencies arising from consolidation. The patient (or surrogate or family) receiving care in the HCO may be expected to act as the intermediary between the billing department of the HCO and the third-party payer, the insurance company, or the MCO. The patient may need to demand referral from the patient's primary-care physician to obtain specialist care. Thus, the patient is expected to help "manage the care" received.

We have looked in some detail at how consolidation can effect board and employees, staff, patients, and the community served by the HCO. If shifts in ownership or alliances of HCOs is going to mean shifts in the values which characterize the ethical climate of the institution, or shifts in the priorities of how the institution operates, people may no longer know what to expect, and may worry that their own role in the institution will change. Consolidation is virtually certain to represent a shift in control such that the balance between cost and quality of care that constitutes the particular character of a given HCO will be less under the control of the internal stakeholders of that HCO. It is inevitable that at least in the short term consolidation will have an adverse effect on the internal ethical climate and the morale of the HCO.

THE ETHICAL CLIMATE OF THE CONTEMPORARY HCO

When we look at the post-1993 HCO, we see an institution that is struggling to accommodate to a number of changes which have been driven by the new emphasis on cost control. The means of achieving the goal of constraining costs is by default primarily market driven, and takes the form of a rapid growth of managed care organizations as intermediaries between the payers and the providers of health care. Unlike earlier MCOs, many contemporary MCOs are not themselves providers of care, but only "managers" of it. The contemporary MCO is a cost-containment, cost-oversight vehicle for employers and government, both of whom have responsibility for the health care of large populations. Many of the new MCOs have their roots in insurance or other commercial enterprises and thus are relatively new to the values that have determined the ethical structure of the HCO. Nevertheless, they will inevitably have an effect on that structure, and on the ethical climate that results.

The HCO has had to react to market forces in order to survive. This reaction has often resulted in some form of consolidation, which itself has resulted in uncertainty and confusion among internal HCO stakeholders. The HCO is being buffeted by change from both within and without.

We have concentrated in this chapter on some of the mechanisms used by MCOs that are particularly troubling in their effect on the HCO and individual provider; but our overall focus on the HCO precludes a more detailed examination of the varieties of managed care. What is clear is that managed care is now the foremost healthcare delivery mechanism in the United States, and is likely to remain so for the foreseeable future. How to address the ethical issues inherent in this system is a major concern, and one that is the responsibility of all elements of the society, not just of the HCO.

Society is beginning to address some of the ethical issues in managed care through legislation, regulation, and other oversight mechanisms. Unfortunately, accrediting bodies and organizations that represent special interests are addressing only particular issues that surface as problematic. The approach is piecemeal and in our view unsatisfactory. For instance, the notorious and short-lived gag rules that were a feature of some MCO contracts prompted legislation in most states as well as proposals being debated on the federal level. The National Committee for Quality Assurance, the primary accrediting body for MCOs in the United States, added a standard for members' rights and responsibilities in 1996 which requires that "members (subscribers to health plans accredited by the organization) have a right to a candid discussion of appropriate or medically necessary treatment options for their condition, regardless of cost or benefit coverage" (NCQA, 1997). In 1997 the newly formed American Association of Healthcare Plans, a group representing the interests of managed care much as the AHA represents the interests of hospitals, developed an initiative called "Putting Patients First" which states that all member plans must adhere to a policy of open disclosure (Jones, 1997). Thus, gag rules have been dealt with but there remain other issues.

MCOs are themselves increasingly aware of the effects of mistrust on their capacity to carry out the functions of oversight and management and perhaps, more importantly, to attract customers. Many are supporting such initiatives as the AAHP Putting Patients First initiative. Such moves, by external accrediting agencies and attempts at self-regulation, may eventually reestablish some of the traditional values in the practices of the MCOs, many of whom, as newcomers, are unaware of the value expectations which have grown up around the vulnerable area of health care. We do not, however, expect any change soon. MCOs will not willingly act in ways which are contrary to their main objective of cost control, and federal and state governments have been unable to articulate the tension that exists between the costs of health care and the quality of health care.

Financial and managerial issues with the objective of cost control will continue to be the driving force behind the changes in the HCO for the foreseeable future. Our concern is with how the HCO can survive the current transitions with its values intact, and how in its interactions with the MCO it can protect those values. Regardless of the cost-control expectations of the HCO, it is still going to be expected to attend to the quality of the care delivered as well. Communication, coordination, and agreement among the different value-producing elements within the HCO will be required to meet both expectations without doing serious damage to the values that constitute the ethical structure of the HCO. We are suggesting the healthcare organization ethics program as a mechanism for that coordination and communication.

If the internal ethical climate of an organization is a function of the perception of its stakeholders as to how well the organization is meeting its expectations of itself (and others' expectations of it), it is not surprising that change, especially rapid change, affects the internal climate negatively. In considering the ethical climate of the contemporary healthcare organization, we are considering a social institution undergoing rapid change. The expectations an organization has of itself, and the expectations its members have of it and of their role within it, are at least in part an artifact of its history. The expectation that an HCO have as its highest priority delivery of high-quality care for a reasonable cost is as old as the history of hospitals in America. But, what is changing is the locus of control about how that responsibility is met.

Clinicians working in the hospitals served the governing board in meeting that expectation in the early years of the republic, defined that expectation in the period between the Civil War and World War II, and collaborated with the board and the administration in the postwar period. It is fair to say that all three periods were characterized by local control. Hospitals were community based. The requirements for high quality care were perceived and evaluated by the people responsible for providing the conditions to meet those requirements, and were in constant view of the community which the hospital served. If shifts in policy or priorities were required, they could be rapid, transparent, and publicly negotiated. Expectations of what the hospital should do were expectations of the people, internal and external to the institution, who were affected by the achievements of the hospital. It was instrumentalities within the hospital—at one time the trustees, later the physicians, most recently administrators—that had the power to structure the institution and the roles of its constituencies or stakeholders in order to accommodate shifts in external expectations and to redefine roles in the institution if necessary to meet those expectations.

The changes that we have been describing in this chapter are disruptive of the power of the HCO to control some of the conditions of healthcare delivery, and they are particularly disruptive of the values that surround health care. If the HCO of tomorrow is to be able to care for the individuals who depend on it, to be worthy of the trust of the society to which it is responsible and the trust of its patients, it needs to create a unified internal ethical climate which can guide decision making and balance institutional priorities.

CONCLUSION

The HCO has the responsibility, whether in a hostile or friendly market environment, to develop and maintain a consistent internal ethical climate. If it takes this responsibility seriously, it will have an influence through its contractual relationships on the ethical climate of those entities with which it does business. It will do this by both implicit and explicit endorsement of those attributes that frame its ethical climate. Building a framework for this internal climate can best be achieved through a process supported by a healthcare organization ethics program. We describe the specifics of such a program in Chapter 9.

8

Developing a Positive Ethical Climate in the Healthcare Organization

In Chapter 7 we concluded that market-based approaches in which health care is viewed as an economic good (Carson, Carson & Roe, 1995, p. 33) have been left, by default, to determine cost, access, and quality. These market-based approaches have resulted in a ferociously competitive environment in which HCOs are struggling for identity as well as survival. The unwillingness of large payers of healthcare benefits to continue to fund increases in the cost of those benefits, combined with ERISA laws and the legal identification of managed care organizations as insurance organizations (which exempts them from antitrust regulations), have given third-party payers and managed care organizations significant negotiating power in their contractual relationships with providers, including HCOs.

HCOs are in the middle of a major shift in the relationships among their stakeholders. Relationships previously viewed by society as sacrosanct—particularly the physician-patient relationship—are significantly affected. Changes in stakeholder relationships have the inevitable effect of changing the internal climate of the HCO.

In the past, explicit societal consensus on changing moral parameters have guided shifts in stakeholder relationships (see Chapter 6), but that is not the case today. Without such a consensus concerning what is permissible in changing our traditions of health care, the result is an ethical climate within the HCO characterized by uncertainty, confusion, and even fear. This unease has also permeated the larger society and has colored the perceptions of the general public and media about HCOs and other institutions involved in the healthcare system.

Ethical initiatives, as well as regulatory responses, have occurred in response to public mistrust. There have been several moves toward self-regulation by the National Committee for Quality Assurance (NCQA), the nation's largest and most prestigious managed care accrediting organization, as well as by the American Association of Health Plans (AAHP), the nation's largest association of managed care plans. We suggested in Chapter 7 that the approach taken by each of these groups is unsatisfactory. Both the NCQA and AAHP react in a piecemeal way to specific problems as these problems attract unfavorable public attention. In our view, neither organization has developed a coherent or comprehensive approach to easing the tensions caused by the widespread imposition of ethically problematic mechanisms (such as capitation) through MCOs' contractual relationships with HCOs and individual providers. Nor have they made any significant effort to educate the public about these arrangements. Furthermore, both organizations represent payer and MCO interests, and it is the early success of the mechanisms MCOs have used to constrain costs that has resulted in the current climate of the HCO. It is unrealistic to expect these organizations to pursue agendas that may put payer and MCO interests in jeopardy especially now, when many experts are predicting increases in insurance premiums (http://www.managedcaremag.com/archiveMC/9903/9903.employer.shtml).

It is equally unrealistic to expect help from federal and state governments. The absence of any explicit discussion leading to a social consensus on the moral parameters within which health care should be delivered leaves governmental bodies equally prey to piecemeal interventions. They, too, have their particular agendas relating to their own costs, employer healthcare costs, patients' satisfaction, and voter perceptions.

The HCO cannot afford to wait for external stakeholders to lead reform initiatives, or to depend upon regulation and legislation to give direction for reform. As the major site for care delivery and for the interaction among payers, providers, and patients, the HCO is in the best position to provide such direction. Our presumption is that one way the HCO can effectively respond to these outside forces is to create a consistent positive internal ethical climate through a fully functioning organization ethics program. This program, through policies and procedures, can help guide stakeholder relationships. A consistent, well-articulated, and well-publicized ethical stance modeled by the HCO can provide an ethical benchmark for both the professionals working in the HCO and the external stakeholders negotiating with it. The ethical standards sustained by the organization ethics program in turn should influence the social environment and provide for the public a model of the moral parameters that should guide the delivery of health care throughout the system.

Developing positive ethical standards within any organization depends on a number of factors. Crucial is the commitment of the leadership of the organization. Equally important is the way in which the strategies, structure, and policies of the organization support its mission. In this chapter, we will first discuss several influences on the development of organization ethics programs. We consider ways to articulate the organization's mission and how they can affect the strategies, structure, and policies of the organization. We consider the impact on both the long-term and day-to-day decision making of the organization's internal climate. In the next chapter we will introduce a detailed model for a healthcare organization ethics process that can be used to address these issues.

THE JCAHO AND ACCREDITATION STANDARDS CONCERNING "ORGANIZATION ETHICS"

As a first step in exploring the potential benefits of developing a consistent internal climate for a HCO, we consider in more detail the opportunity presented by the Joint Commission for Accreditation of Health Care Organizations' requirements for an "organization ethics function." In 1995 the JCAHO added a section called "Organization Ethics" to its Standards for Patient Rights and Ethics. This focused the attention of the healthcare organizations it accredits on a particular set of issues that had not yet been addressed by other healthcare industry regulatory mechanisms. By requiring attention to these issues, the JCAHO explicitly recognized that organizational structures have the clear potential to affect patient care.

The JCAHO addresses the organization ethics function under five headings: conduct and conflict, code of ethics, organs, research, and managing staff requests. The two subgroups that we are most concerned with, code of ethics and conduct and conflict, require an examination of a number of specific activities and relationships within the organization. These activities include disclosure of referral services, contracts, marketing, admission, transfer, discharge, and billing practices, as well as the relationship of the hospital and its staff members to other healthcare providers, educational institutions, and payers. An appropriate examination of these activities requires (1) knowing what the current policies are; and (2) knowing what influence these policies have on activities as they are actually carried out. The JCAHO is, in effect, asking each HCO that it accredits to consider whether its actual activities are compatible with its stated vision of itself. Whether its standards are represented in the long-run decisions the HCO makes or in the day-to-day decisions made by and on behalf of HCO stakeholders is an expression of the HCO's internal ethical climate.

As we suggested in Chapter 1, there are some limitations to the JCAHO's definition of healthcare organization ethics. Their definition includes all activities of the organization that currently affect patient care, and it requires attention to particular relationships which the HCO may have within this context. It does not, however, address the possibility that the overall ethical climate of the organization may be influenced by policies and activities that do not have a direct patient care orientation; nor does it address how this ethical climate can be developed and maintained. Further, the JCAHO definition is not specifically concerned with those issues that may arise in the HCO's relation to managed care organizations, government entities, employers, and insurance companies. As an alternative to the JCAHO definition, we called attention to the more comprehensive definition advanced by the Virginia Bioethics Network, which states, "Organization ethics consists of a process(es) to address ethical issues associated with the business, financial, and management areas of healthcare organizations, as well as with professional, educational, and contractual relationships affecting the operation of the HCO" (see Appendix 1).

The JCAHO itself has already begun to expand the scope of its initial Organization Ethics Standards. It understands that HCOs cannot formulate a functional code of ethics without attention to the core values that are presumed in *all* HCO stakeholder relationships. In the 1997 Comprehensive Accreditation Manual for Hospitals, the following was added:

> RI.4.1.1 The hospital's code of ethical business and professional behavior protects the integrity of clinical decision-making, regardless of how the hospital shares financial risk with its leaders, managers, clinical staff, and licensed independent practitioners.
>
> Intent of RI.4.1.1 To avoid compromising the quality of care, clinical decisions, including tests, treatments and other interventions, are based on identified patient healthcare needs. The hospital's code of ethical business and professional behavior specifies that the hospital implements policies and procedures that address this issue. Policies and procedures and information about the relationship between the use of services and financial incentives are available on request to all patients, clinical staff, licensed independent practitioners and hospital personnel.

While the JCAHO does not explicitly address what we defined as the HCO's ethical climate, it makes clear that the integrity of clinical ethical decision making must be a core value of the HCO and that this particular core value must receive ongoing attention by the HCO. Further, the JCAHO has also made it clear through Intent of RI.4.1.1 that having an organization code of ethics is not enough. The JCAHO requires that the institution operate within this code by supporting it with policies and procedures that can guide decision making. The code itself simply provides an outline of how the institution will ensure ethical operation, and this outline is to be expanded within each HCO by appropriate internal policy development.

The JCAHO has provided an accredited HCO the opportunity to look closely at itself—at its values and mission, and the way by which it intends to consider its values and fulfill its mission. The JCAHO has not dictated how exactly the HCO should approach this opportunity, nor has it stated any requirements for its implementation. It has, however, identified one core value that it believes is nonnegotiable in health care: the integrity of clinical decision making. It has left the way open for the HCO to identify other core values.

HCO RESPONSE TO CHANGING ACCREDITATION REQUIREMENTS

Response to the JCAHO Organizational Ethics Standards has varied, but many HCOs have tried to form an organization ethics program that not only will respond to these standards, but also will truly attempt to develop and articulate strategies, policies, and procedures that will produce or enhance a consistent positive ethical climate for the entire organization. To our knowledge these efforts, even in the most committed organizations, are in their early stages and their ultimate success or failure cannot yet be known. However, we are optimistic concerning the likely success of these efforts and believe this full-hearted response should be the goal of each HCO.

Many other HCOs have approached the JCAHO Organizational Ethics Standards with a wait-and-see attitude. They understand that some past JCAHO standards have had to be modified or dropped because they were not applicable or sustainable in the real world of healthcare delivery. Before attempting to commit employee time and other resources to organization ethics development, they do only what is necessary to pass JCAHO inspections. A third group of HCOs is attempting to fulfill only the minimum requirements of the JCAHO Organization Ethics Standards by developing the required code of ethics that addresses, on paper, each of the issues listed by the JCAHO. It is possible to do that while doing next to nothing to make the code a meaningful set of goals for the organization, but to do so is to miss an opportunity to address many of the wider issues that face the HCO.

As noted in Chapter 1, the American Hospital Association (AHA) has developed an organization ethics initiative. All indications are that it plans to require that each of its member organizations (essentially all U.S. hospitals) have an organization ethics program. It has somewhat stringent requirements as to what must be addressed by this program. With both the AHA and the JCAHO paying increasing attention to organization ethics as a very important aspect of the overall goals and operations of the HCO, it is becoming essentially mandatory for each HCO to develop and support an organization ethics program and to begin this development process now.

LEADERSHIP IN THE HCO

One important element in organization effectiveness is leadership. Tom Peters and Robert H. Waterman in their groundbreaking book *In Search of Excellence* rather ruefully admit that they kept coming back to the idea of leadership in their search for what made a company excellent. Peters and Waterman argue that it is shared values that make an organization effective, but that "in almost every excellent company was a strong leader (or two) who seemed to have had a lot to do with making the company excellent in the first place. Many of these companies—for instance, IBM, P&G [Procter and Gamble], Emerson, J&J [Johnson and Johnson], and Dana—seem to have taken on their basic character under the tutelage of a very special person. Moreover, they did it at a fairly early stage in their development" (Peters & Waterman, 1982, p. 26).

This theme of leadership supplying the vision and articulating the values of an organization consistently surfaces in management discussions and research. (Treviño et al., 1999; Montoya & Richard, 1994, p. 714). The point is not that one or two leaders make the organization effective, but that leadership articulates and defines the organization's values, which when committed to by the leadership allows them to be shared throughout the organization. This allows the organization to be effective.

Treviño et al. discuss the role of top management in contributing to a positive ethical climate within the organization. It is the commitment of the CEO and other leaders that renew the values of the organization and determine the ethical tone of the organization (Treviño et al., 1999, p. 141). It is the example and commitment of leadership to a positive ethical climate in an organization that engenders positive outcomes like employee awareness of ethical or legal issues, reporting bad news to management, reporting ethical or legal violations, refraining from unethical or illegal conduct, higher employee commitment to the organization, and the belief among employees that decision making is better (p. 139).

But leadership in HCOs has not until now needed to examine the internal ethical climate of their organization or provide an articulated vision of the HCO's values. Until recently, HCOs have enjoyed generous government funding and third-party reimbursement policies. Historically, HCO leadership has accepted the values within which society has believed health care should be delivered.

Although diverse groups have provided leadership in the HCO through various periods, with power shifting to one group or another depending on shifting societal values, these groups (administrators, physicians, and governing boards) were not subjected to competing and mutually exclusive goals. Each group was able to achieve the goals expected of it without having to sacrifice in any meaningful way the goals of other groups. Because competitive pressures were absent, supportive and collaborative relations between groups of internal stakeholders were possible.

So it was that many HCOs, until the death of the Clinton plan, could be called excellent in terms of sharing with their stakeholders a strong sense of values endorsed by the community along with a commitment to those values—and HCOs were thereby living up to society's values. As we argued in Chapter 7, this is no longer the case. Control of health care threatens to move outside the institution and into the hands of the various mediators between the patient and payers for the care received by the patient.

Top management helps develop, articulate, and support the values the organization uses as a basis for its policies and day-to-day procedures. It should provide consistent examples of how the organization carries out its mission in a positive ethical manner. But as we made clear in the previous chapter, pressures abound for that leadership to be divisive and uncertain. Today's HCO leadership must struggle with cost-containment measures that could put the organization in financial jeopardy. It must implement ethically problematic mechanisms that achieve cost-containment goals by constraining relationships among important HCO stakeholders, including patients and the professional staff, and which threaten the collaborative efforts of the past. It must make decisions and choices that were once inconceivable, and it must do so in the absence of clearly understood and endorsed societal values.

ARTICULATING VALUES AND STANDARDS

Ethical standards or values espoused by organizations are generally articulated in mission statements, value statements, vision statements, or codes of ethics. These core organization values represent how the organization perceives of itself as an ethical entity, distinguishes the organization from other organizations, are relatively enduring over time, and influence both the structure of the organization and the roles and behavior of stakeholders in the organization (Forehand & Gilmer, 1964).

Mission statements, values statements, vision statements, or codes of ethics are forms of expression used by organizations to address questions of what the organization does, what values it subscribes to in carrying out its central purpose, and where the organization wants to be at sometime in the future. Organizations often label these statements interchangeably, making it sometimes difficult to specify which statement describes which issue or activity—one organization's value statement may be another's mission statement. However, no matter how they are labeled in a particular HCO, the core values found in these statements should form the underlying framework for the articulation of the organization's internal ethical climate. These statements express the ethical standards by which the organization wishes to be judged. But these statements in themselves are not sufficient to understand the organization's ethical climate. Statements are just that—statements. Policies and day-to-day activities based on the common expectations of particular responses are the best indication of how well the organization lives up to its vision of itself as defined in its vision or value statements.

It is important, however, to understand that these statements can combine operational or applied elements with philosophical or core value elements (Darr,

1997). This distinction is valid since core values distinguish the organization; they endure, even though operational elements may change over time in response to internal or external changes. Consider for instance portions of the mission statement of St. Mary's Hospital, located in Huntington, West Virginia, and note the combination of core values, the values the organization prioritizes, and operational elements that describe the scope of its activities:

> Respecting the God-given dignity of each person, we continually strive to improve the quality of our service. We wish to deliver it in ways which are responsive to the health needs of our community, with a special concern for the poor, and in ways which manifest the values of compassion, hospitality, reverence, interdependence, stewardship, and trust.

This portion of St. Mary's mission statement contains an explicit commitment to the organization's core values of compassion, hospitality, reverence, interdependence, stewardship, and trust. Operational elements are found in the following portion of St. Mary's mission statement:

> The Hospital provides acute, skilled nursing, and home health services for persons . . . by offering a broad range of primary and specialty health services for inpatients, outpatients and patients in their homes. (http://www.st-marys.org/mission.html)

In the above example St. Mary's core values of compassion, hospitality, reverence, interdependence, stewardship and trust need not change even if portions of St. Mary's operational elements change (e.g., if St. Mary's discontinued home health services.)

Core values articulated by organizations may occasionally lead to conflicts of commitment. In Chapter 5 we discussed professional conflicts of interest and mentioned conflicts of commitment in individual professionals as mainly role conflicts. Organizations, too, face conflicts of interest and conflicts of commitment. Conflicts of interest and commitment occur in organizations where organizational demands conflict with its mission. If the mission of a HCO states that it provides health care for a defined population, then limited resources place it in an almost perpetual conflict-of-commitment situation. An HCO that allegedly exists to serve patients, yet prioritizes profitability, places itself and its managers in a conflict of commitment. Such an organizational culture usually creates conflicts of commitment for professionals in the organization as well.

Interestingly, in HCOs most conflicts of this sort are best defined as conflicts of commitment, not conflicts of interest. Because every HCO has to find means to be economically viable, conflicts between that commitment and commitments to provide health care inevitably clash, even in HCOs that prioritize patient care as their primary mission. Without infinite resources, HCOs cannot provide every kind of health care to every one of their patients, nor can most HCOs adequately serve the uninsured population. These are not merely conflicts of interest, because they require choosing between two specific stated (or unstated but recognized) commitments of the HCO based on conflicting core values.

Many of these conflicts cannot be avoided. However, there are steps an organization can take to mitigate the effects of the conflicts. The most important of these steps revolve around early recognition of conflict situations and full disclosure of the conflicts to all stakeholders who may be negatively affected by the conflicts in question. Other strategies for dealing with conflicts of interest and conflicts of commitment include:

1. Disclosure and publicity are essential elements. Stakeholders, whether they are patients, professionals, or managers who are aware of conflicting organizational demands and capabilities are much more understanding of organizational conflicts and the difficulty in resolving all of them to the satisfaction of everyone involved.
2. Performing "triage" on commitments: prioritizing them in terms of who is least harmed or most benefited, which demands are necessary for organizational excellence, which most emulate organizational mission, which least violate one's other role commitments, and which can be put aside.
3. Perform "organizational self-assessment" for structures or accountability procedures that create conflicts of commitment. One needs to trace the origins of the conflicts and address these structural problems if they are evident as part of the cause of conflict.

We envision that the organization ethics process, described in the next chapter, will provide a mechanism so that conflict resolution between stakeholders, between individuals and systems, and between stakeholders (including organizations) and the HCO, can be facilitated within the context of organizations' internal ethical climate represented by their stated core values.

CORE VALUES AND ORGANIZATIONAL WELL-BEING

The healthcare industry is widely perceived as becoming a for-profit business rather than providing a valued social function, and the perceived credo of for-profits has been maximization of shareholder return. But even nonprofit HCOs cannot survive without an appropriate return on their assets. An HCO must have sufficient operating capital for its maintenance needs, and it must be in a strong enough financial position to obtain funds to invest in new technology or exploit growth opportunities. This is true for all organizations that exist to provide a product or a service. Does an organizational commitment to a core value—like community service—imply that the HCO will not be able to survive in a highly competitive market? That it will squander a competitive advantage or waste precious resources? As mentioned above, there is increasing evidence that a competitive advantage is actually *formed* by a commitment to core values.

In a six-year project James Collins and Jerry Porras set out to identify and systematically research the historical development of a set of what they called visionary companies, to examine how these companies differed from a carefully selected control set of comparison companies (Collins & Porras, 1994, p. 2). Their interest lay in explaining the enduring quality and prosperity of these visionary companies.

Collins and Porras defined the visionary company as the premier organization in its industry, as being widely admired by its peers, and as having a long track record of making a significant impact on the world around it. The companies identified by Collins and Porras included 3M, American Express, Boeing, Citicorp, Ford, General Electric, Hewlett-Packard, IBM, Johnson and Johnson, Marriott, Merck, Motorola, Nordstrom, Phillip Morris, Procter & Gamble, Sony, Wal-Mart, and Walt Disney. Each of the visionary companies chosen had faced setbacks; each had made mistakes but each had displayed a resiliency, an ability to bounce back from adversity. The long-run performance of each has been remarkable. A dollar invested in a visionary company stock fund on January 1, 1926, with dividends reinvested, and making appropriate adjustments for when the companies became available on the stock market would have grown by December 31, 1990, to $6,356. That dollar invested in a general market fund would have grown to only $415 (p. 5).

The comparison companies chosen by Collins and Porras are by no means sluggards. They represent some of the most respected organizations in the world. They include Ames, Burroughs, Bristol-Myers, Chase, Colgate, Columbia, General Motors, Howard Johnson, Kenwood, McDonnell Douglas, Norton, Pfizer, R.J. Reynolds, Texas Instruments, Wells Fargo, Westinghouse, and Zenith. That dollar invested in a comparison stock fund composed of these companies would have returned $955— more than twice the general market but less than one-sixth of the return provided by the visionary companies (p. 5).

What was different about visionary companies and comparison companies? Both operated in the same market and each had relatively the same opportunities. What was it that allowed a visionary company to endure setbacks, compete successfully in markets that are just as difficult as the one currently faced by the HCO, and overcome, on occasion, strategic decisions that threatened the very existence of the organization?

Collins and Porras exploded a number of myths in the course of their research, including the myth that insists that the most successful companies exist first and foremost to maximize profits:

> Contrary to business school doctrine, "maximizing shareholder wealth" or "profit maximization" has not been the dominant driving force or primary objective through

> the history of the visionary companies. Visionary companies pursue a cluster of objectives, of which making money is only one—and not necessarily the primary one. Yes, they seek profits, but they are equally guided by a core ideology—core values and a sense of purpose beyond just making money. Yet, paradoxically, the visionary companies make more money than the more purely profit-driven comparison companies. (p. 8)

Collins and Porras found that lucky breaks, or great product ideas, or market insights, or "great and charismatic" leadership of the "high-profile" type could not explain visionary companies. Visionary companies displayed an organization-wide commitment to their stated core values and a sense of purpose in realizing their missions. This commitment and sense of purpose translate into enduring prosperity. These conclusions suggest a model for HCOs. If one takes as the primary mission of the HCO patient or population health care, and if that mission forms the core value that the organization sees as its vision and source of direction despite the vicissitudes of markets, regulation, public policy, or other environmental changes, then that organization will be able to survive and even flourish in the chaos of a changing healthcare system. Moreover, by focusing on a central core mission, the question of profitability, when properly prioritized near the bottom of the list of goals, is no longer an overriding issue.

Although the findings of Collins and Porras may seem to refute the contention of Peters and Waterman that excellent companies almost always had one or more identifiable strong leaders, on closer examination the findings of these two groups are fully compatible and not antagonistic. Peters and Waterman also stressed the primary importance of a unique set of shared values as a prerequisite for excellence, but noted the importance of strong leadership in articulating and maintaining these values. Collins and Porras do not dispute that organization effectiveness depends on the leadership of the organization. Their concern is in explaining that organizations need not have a "great and charismatic" leader to be visionary. Visionary companies may not have high-profile leadership, but they do have leadership that is committed to the core values of the organization. Later we shall suggest that a well-positioned organization ethics committee could serve in such a leadership capacity.

STRATEGIES AND STRUCTURE

The operational or applied elements of the mission statements, values statements, vision statements, or codes of ethics will answer questions of what the organization does, what it wants to do, and what it will do to get there.

These operational elements are the result of high-level decisions that are often referred to as "corporate strategies." A corporate strategy is the result of a process that seeks to monitor and adjust to changes in the organization's environment within the framework of the organization's mission (Krajewski & Ritzman, 1993). Corporate strategies have a long-term horizon and tend to be inseparably linked to the mission of the organization because they require major commitments of present and future resources. Corporate strategies result in decisions concerning organizational growth, retrenchment, or stability (Carson, Carson & Roe, 1995). These considerations are linked to the survival of the organization.

Corporate strategies should be framed within the context of the organization's core values because corporate strategies are the practical reflection of the organization's vision of itself. If, for example, an HCO has made an explicit commitment to the community that it serves, it should consider the effect on the community of discontinuing an existing service. If corporate strategies are framed within the context of the organization's core values, then management will have little trouble translating those core values into the next layer of strategy, sometimes called the "business" or "tactical" strategy. This is the practical adaptation of the "corporate strategy." This lower-level strategy focuses on how the corporate strategy can be achieved. It is detail oriented and specifies the tasks that the organization must accomplish within certain time frames in order to support the longer-term corporate strategy. Again, it should be noted that even though this is a shorter-term strategy designed to achieve specific goals it should reflect the organization's commitment to its values.

In the previous example, St. Mary's states that they wish to deliver healthcare services in ways that are responsive to the health needs of their community. If this is their vision of themselves, their corporate strategy will adjust to changes in the community and St. Mary's will consider offering new services or discontinuing old services depending on changes in the community they serve. This may involve capital expenditures on technology and buildings. These decisions have the potential to determine St. Mary's survival.

Their business strategies will reflect this long-term commitment; while most shorter-term strategies may not affect the long-term survival of St. Mary's, they should be designed within the context of both St. Mary's vision of itself and its long-term corporate strategy. For instance, St. Mary's might well begin to adjust its employment profiles depending on the services it sees itself offering in the future. However, if St. Mary's is serious about its core values, both strategies will reflect concern for the poor, and manifest the values of compassion, hospitality, reverence, interdependence, stewardship, and trust.

Both corporate and business strategies affect the structure of the organization (defined here as the resources in place to support existing activities). For instance, if the HCO's long-term strategy is growth through diversification of services offered, and the business strategy consists of decisions on how best to achieve this objective, the structure of the organization will reflect these strategies. Such questions concerning structure as the following may be important: If the HCO needs to add additional prenatal activities to expand its services, can its existing structure accommodate the change or should an entirely new clinic be set up? What new technology may be required? What will be needed to support it? Will the organization require different skills from its employees? Will it require new employees? How is success defined? How will the organization monitor the new activity to ensure its success? Answers to these questions may change the organization's existing structure. *But it is through the structure the organization employs, including the policies that support this structure that most interactions among its stakeholders occur.* These interactions form the basis for perceptions of stakeholders, both internal and external, as to whether the organization means what it says. For instance, the hospital's stated values reflect concern and compassion for the poor. If the poor interact with St. Mary's structures through the emergency room and various clinics and the poor are not shown compassion, respect, and caring, then both the poor of the community and St. Mary's staff understand that a gap exists between St. Mary's stated values and its actual values.

If the core values of the organization are reflected at all levels of organizational strategies, then they will be reflected in whatever structural changes or day-to-day policies the organization employs to realize its vision of itself. The organization, which has identified and articulated values it is committed to and is serious about promoting these values to both its internal and external stakeholders, will find that changes or shifts in business strategies will not necessarily have a major effect on the organization's internal ethical climate. For instance, in the St. Mary's example above, the core value of concern for the poor need not change even if St. Mary's must discontinue a previously offered service. It is simply that St. Mary's develops a different structure in order to realize this value as conditions in the community it serves change.

POLICIES

Policies are the link between the mission and vision of the organization and its strategies and structure. They manifest themselves in the practical application of these mandates and guidelines in planning and in everyday practice. Generally, policies are formulated at the very top of the organization and may be presented as guidelines or they may be precise. Consider the following example:

Eastern Mercy Health System, based in Radnor, Pennsylvania, is sponsored by nine regional Communities of the Sisters of Mercy and includes sixteen acute-care hospitals and twenty other facilities in seven eastern states. Mercy is the seventh largest not-for-profit health system in the country, operating in five states. This system endorses three principles:

1. Respect for the dignity of the human person
2. Dignity can only be protected and realized in community
3. Special responsibility for the poor

The result of the practical application of these principles was an eight-page docu-ment called "Ethical Guidelines for Managed Care." These guidelines were pub-lished in June 1995, and after a four-month pilot at four institutions, were distrib-uted to executives in the system who are responsible for negotiating contracts with managed care organizations.

The document links guidance on various issues to the principles to which the organization is committed. It is prescriptive on some issues, for instance, insur-ing that the needs of the poor and underserved are addressed, and nonnegotiable on others, for instance abortion. The document has received favorable notices from system executives who view the document as a tool which can avoid misunder-standings and which provides a framework for negotiation (Appleby, 1996). In this manner Eastern Mercy Health System has helped ensure control of its own destiny by consistently applying its values not only within its system but also to its external partners through contractual mandates.

The articulation of an organization's core values through its policies is intended to have, and within organizations that take them seriously does have, a profound effect on the strategics and structure of an organization. Policies help tie together mission and vision statements and corporate structure and strategies and ensure that the strategies and structures employed by the organization to fulfill its mis-sion will exist within the context of the organization's core values.

CONCLUSION

Our concern in this chapter has been to discuss some of the important elements that affect the internal ethical climate of healthcare organizations. These elements include the leadership of the organization, the vision, mission, and values of the organization, the organization's strategies and structure, and the translation of the organization's core values into policies that can guide the organization through both the long and the short term.

We have supplied evidence (Chapter 7) to support our observation that the in-ternal climate of the HCO is in need of repair. We have argued that HCOs should not view an examination of the elements that make up an organization's internal climate as an exercise in expending resources for which there will be little or no return. We cited research that supports the contention that organizations that in-vest their core values with a sense of purpose are the most enduring and prosper-ous organizations in the world.

We have also suggested that the organization ethics standards promulgated by the JCAHO should be viewed as an opportunity that will enable the HCO to set the moral parameters within which health care is delivered. It is an opportunity for the HCO to define itself within its mission and its vision of itself. If this op-portunity is seized, the HCO can do more than just influence or develop its own internal climate—it can affect the external climate in which health care is delivered as well.

The elements discussed in this chapter, since they are associated with the efficient and effective operation of all types of organizations, of necessity will be an important aspect of the planning and implementation of an organization ethics program for a HCO. In the next chapter we flesh out our concept of what an organization ethics program should be. We call attention to the policies the HCO should begin to examine or formulate as it considers the direction for its organization ethics process. A healthcare organization ethics process is described in detail and advanced as the mechanism by which the HCO can address conflicts of interest and conflicts of commitments.

9

Instituting an Organization Ethics Program

In chapter 8 we discussed the role of the mission statement, value statement, or ethical code in the HCO. These represent the vehicle for introducing central ethical content into the HCO. Long- and short-term organizational strategies and structures need to be formulated with these values in mind. It is the ethical standards expressed in the mission statement that the organization ethics program aims to implement throughout the institution.

But merely to state ethical values is not sufficient. As we concluded in Chapters 1 through 5, the HCO itself is best understood as a dynamic set of structures, processes, and activities in constant interaction with its internal and external environment. Maintaining positive ethical standards in such an open system is itself a task that requires a flexible, informed, active, ongoing implementation and oversight process. It is the details of setting up such a process through the development of an organization ethics committee that this chapter addresses.

How does one develop an organization ethics program? Such a program must take into account the complex relationships between all the HCO stakeholders, respect professional excellence and managerial expertise, and deal with clinical and compliance issues—all while encouraging a positive ethical climate within the organization conducive to the delivery of excellent patient care.

Developing an organization ethics program involves self-study and the appointment of an organization ethics development team. The development team will be responsible for tailoring their recommendations to the requirements and resources of the institution, determining what role the program should play in the HCO and what its activities should be, and making recommendations to the governing board.

A logical first step is to study the HCO's status in relation to its mission and core values, and to determine what structures and activities are the major determinants of its ethical climate. Every HCO should have, or should develop, a clearly articulated mission statement. Throughout this book we have argued that the primary mission of a healthcare organization, by definition, is to provide adequate health care to its patients or to a defined population. This mission is derived from the traditional role of hospitals, and remains central to what our society expects from healthcare organizations. Such a mission does not preclude profitability, but it prioritizes patient care and the professional excellence necessary to provide adequate care as primary goals. In laying out mechanisms for instituting a comprehensive organization ethics program, we assume that an HCO already has, or will develop, a mission statement modeled after these priorities. If an HCO has different priorities, those should be articulated and publicly justified.

If there is a mission statement, value statement, or code of ethics in place, it may be useful to study the present ethical climate of the organization in order to establish a baseline for any improvements. Some suggestions for studying the climate are found in Chapter 11. Following the articulation of the mission and a study of the perceived ethical climate of the organization, recommendations for needed changes must be developed and ultimately made to the governing board. These recommendations will concern the specifics of the development of a meaningful and effective organization ethics program, one that will articulate the organization's ethical climate via mission statement, core values, code of ethics, and policy criteria. Most importantly, the program will need to develop an ongoing education-and-enhancement program that will integrate the organization's mission into all activities, and at all levels, from the governing board to the maintenance staff.

Development of appropriate recommendations for the HCO's governing board can best be accomplished by the appointment of an organization ethics planning or development team. After appropriate study of the pertinent issues, it will make recommendations for needed changes to the governing board. The importance of the work of this team can not be overstated, so recruitment of appropriate members is paramount. Membership should represent all of the major areas and departments of the HCO, and each member should have an interest in the development of the organization ethics program. The administration, the clinical professions, the legal department, the patient care ethics committee, and the governing board itself should be represented on the organization ethics development team.

The organization ethics development team must have a clear mandate from the governing board or administration. We emphasized the importance of leadership in the previous chapter; and the organization ethics program cannot be successful in its task unless it is supported from the highest level. Each team member must be aware of the importance of his task in structuring the program so as to assure its success in the particular HCO.

Recommendations from the planning group are of critical importance, and specific issues that should be addressed during the planning process include:

1. Will compliance and accreditation activities be subsumed under the organization ethics program?
2. Where does the organization ethics program fit into the administrative structure?
3. Will patient care ethics activities be addressed by the program?
4. How and to what extent will professional ethics issues be addressed by the program?
5. Should the program be advisory only, or should it have limited (or extended) decision-making authority?
6. Will the program have the authority to influence decisions concerning contractual relationships of the HCO to other entities that do not adhere to the same moral ground rules as the HCO itself?
7. Finally, how should the program itself be structured?

We will address each of these questions in the sections that follow.

WILL COMPLIANCE OR ACCREDITATION ACTIVITIES BE ADDRESSED BY THE ORGANIZATION ETHICS PROGRAM?

There have been two major stimuli leading to the institution of organization ethics programs. One has been Justice Department attention and the perceived need for a government-approved compliance program. The other has been the JCAHO's promulgation of standards addressing organization ethics issues. How to respond to these compliance and accreditation requirements has been a major concern in most HCOs.

Many HCOs have seen the organization ethics requirements of the JCAHO and the necessity to have a mechanism to address federal compliance as separate issues. These HCOs have two distinct committees or working groups with separate missions or goals. The compliance committee (or officer) narrowly addresses compliance with federal laws and regulations, since to do so, according to the Federal Sentencing Guidelines, can mitigate potential sentences (as we discuss in more detail in Chapter 10). The organization ethics committee or subcommittee is a more recent innovation that has been instituted to meet the JCAHO standards for an organization code of ethics and supporting policies and procedures. This two-pronged approach often ignores consideration of the larger issue of what each of these activities means for an HCO which is attempting to define itself ethically. Although using two separate groups to focus on these particular issues may fulfill the letter of the law for both the federal government and the JCAHO, we believe attention to these issues is better accomplished under a single umbrella committee. This pathway for attention to accreditation and compliance issues within an HCO is one that should serve the HCO better than two committees working on similar issues but with separate agendas.

A comprehensive organization ethics program that adequately addresses the mission, activities, and ethical climate of the HCO, should completely fulfill the JCAHO accreditation requirements, particularly if the program includes the development of an organization code of ethics that address the specific issues the JCAHO requires: marketing, admission, transfer, discharge, billing practices, providers, payers, and educational institutions. There are good reasons to include all of the JCAHO accreditation requirements for organization ethics under the mandate for the HCO's organization ethics program, and few if any reasons not to include them. Inclusion of JCAHO requirements in the organization ethics program prevents duplication of efforts and possible dilution of the authority of the program itself.

The relation of compliance programs to the organization ethics program is not a simple matter, and we discuss it at several places in this book. We argue in Chapter 10 that organization ethics functions should not be subsumed under the compliance program. In this chapter we suggest that the converse is not true. Some compliance activities can be a component of the organization ethics program, if some conditions are met. The advantages of having compliance as one component or subcommittee of the larger organization ethics process include communication between sometimes compartmentalized groups, and early warning of legal threats to ethical integrity.

Specific compliance activities that meet federal standards and therefore qualify as grounds for the mitigation of required sentences are spelled out in the Federal Sentencing Guidelines. Many of the issues covered by those activities should be considered by the organization ethics program as well, and can be specified as such in the policies under which the program operates. The legal compliance of an HCO, like its compliance to high standards of ethics, is one of the normative considerations that determines the ethical climate of an organization. As we suggested in Chapter 2, the relation of ethics and law is not a simple one. In many cases, law and regulation are imposed to force compliance to ethical standards. We assume that strict attention to ethical issues can effectively meet, and often exceeds, legal requirements. If the organization ethics committee takes seriously its mandate to integrate ethics throughout the organization, it will cover many of the same activities as the compliance program, and can contribute to its effective functioning.

There are some activities required for an approved compliance program, such as the monitoring of auditing systems designed to detect criminal behavior, that appear not to fit into the activities to be expected of an organization ethics program. However, the goal of the compliance program is at least congruent with the overall goal of the organization ethics program, particularly if the organization ethics program is seen as the area within the HCO for oversight of ethical issues of all types. To grant this inclusive mandate to the organization ethics program would give it authority to consider those legal issues which are directly associated with noncompliance to particular laws or regulations, and should allow for development of appropriate methods for consideration of compliance issues which are not strictly defined as ethical issues or processes related to ethical issues.

To be an effective purveyor and guardian of the HCO's ethical climate, an organization ethics program should not only meet the demands of the JCAHO guidelines, but also be a potent ally of the compliance program. Those accreditation activities which are required in JCAHO organization ethics standards and some institutional activities required for compliance with governmental regulations will be addressed by a comprehensive organization ethics program.

WHERE DOES AN ORGANIZATION ETHICS PROGRAM FIT INTO THE HCO'S ADMINISTRATIVE STRUCTURE?

One of the first issues to be addressed by the organization ethics planning committee is the administrative location of the program. This decision may well be the most important decision for assuring the effectiveness of the organization ethics program or, conversely, in assuring that it will have difficulty in meeting its stated objectives. In order to be maximally effective, the organization ethics program must meet several conditions. It must have respect; it must be visible throughout the organization; and it must be vested with some degree of authority.

The task of the organization ethics program is to align all organizational activities with the mission and ethical standards of the organization. This task is important to organizational success in terms of morale, reputation, and competitive advantage; its success will contribute to the cohesiveness and integration of the HCO. In order to gain and retain the respect of both internal and external stakeholders, it is crucial that the program not be seen as in the service of specific departmental agendas, or have its decisions and recommendations subordinated to any goals other than responsibility for the ethical climate. It cannot succeed without the trust of the organization at all levels, and it cannot gain and keep this trust without behaving responsibly to its primary function.

The program cannot be used, or be useful, if it is invisible, compartmentalized, or inaccessible to large numbers of its constituents. Its role in the institution needs to be widely understood, and it needs to constantly monitor its effectiveness in the eyes of its constituents. Both communication and education are central to establishing the necessary high profile within the organization.

Maintaining high ethical standards in times of rapid change can require flex-ibility, innovation, and responsiveness. Decisions about marketing, admission or billing practices, long- or short-term strategic considerations, or contracts with suppliers and payers can all have consequences which resonate throughout the institution, affecting clinicians or requiring structural change. The program will need timely access to information about what is happening in the organization, and authority to address issues which will affect either adherence to ethical stan-dards or stakeholder perceptions of that adherence. All these considerations lead to the conclusion that the administrative location of the organization ethics pro-gram needs to be at a high level within the HCO.

There are several alternatives of where to administratively locate the organiza-tion ethics program. We shall consider each in turn.

HCO administration

Because of the desirability of maintaining a focus on the JCAHO standards, de-velopment teams may recommend that the organization ethics program should consist of administrators, legal advisors, finance officers, risk managers, plus one or more board members. Some may recommend inclusion of representatives from the professional staff, but many will not.

If organized in this manner, the organization ethics program will basically be a responsibility of the HCO's administration and therefore have an administrative perspective. If it reports to the CEO the organization ethics program has the op-portunity to affect organizational decision making at the highest levels and can have the authority it needs to have an impact on the organization as a whole. However, we believe that locating the organization ethics program as a direct function of the administration would be a mistake. The CEO and other adminis-trators may have obligations that are not congruent with the organization's over-all mission in particular situations. It is the role of top-level management to con-sider the organization's mission and how this relates to financial well-being and strategic positioning, and to consider as well the constraints the organization con-fronts in achieving its mission. There will inevitably be circumstances in which maintaining a positive ethical climate consistent with the mission of the organi-zation is seen as a constraint on the processes that the administration must con-sider in fulfilling its obligations. There may be a natural tendency for the admin-istration to attempt to bypass or ignore the implications of a decision that reinforces the mission and improves the ethical climate of the organization, but harms its financial well-being. Moreover, without professional and patient representation an organization ethics program fails in its mandate to represent the primary stake-holders of the HCO. Therefore, while it is crucial that the organization ethics pro-gram has access to, and be supported by top administration, it is not desirable for it to be, or be perceived to be, a purely administrative function.

Legal department

Both JCAHO standards and federal compliance standards address issues central to an HCO's ethical climate, issues such as proper disclosure, conflicts of interest and conflicts of commitment, confidentiality, payment mechanisms, contractual relationships with healthcare professionals, and contractual relationships with other individuals and organizations. These issues, and the internal and external processes related to them, are also either directly or indirectly the responsibility of the HCO's legal department. This raises the obvious question, should the organization ethics program be administratively located in the legal department?

Just as it is the role of top level administration to consider first and foremost the organization's financial well-being, legal advisors have an obligation to protect the organization from risk of loss from legal liability, either from lack of compliance to laws and regulations, or from the potential for an adverse outcome in a particular law suit. There will be times when requirements for full legal protection may be antagonistic to the mandates required by the organizational mission and maintained by the organization ethics program. For example, suppose that a major mistake has been made in medicating a patient directly leading to her death. There is no likely way for the family of the patient to discover that the mistake resulted in the death. Some legal advisors might suggest that the incident not be disclosed since there is no real remedy and appropriate measures have been taken to address the problem that led to the mistake. If the HCO espouses honest disclosure as a part of its core values or code of ethics and this conflicts with the mandate of the legal department, the organization ethics program should be in a position to consider both claims, rather than be administratively subordinated to one of the claimants.

The legal department is frequently the source of mandates that may be necessary to protect the organization but do nothing to enhance its ethical climate. Further, many features of the contemporary situation which make an organization ethics program desirable are a function of changes where the law is silent, inapplicable, or lagging behind social need. Legal mandates tend to be constraining and based only on present-day law, while the organization ethics program's interests are broader, preventative rather than reactive, and more open. Locating the organization ethics program in the legal department enhances the perception that it is mainly a compliance, quality assurance, and public relations activity and appears to have no real authority to openly address disputed ethical positions, some of which may be contrary to the mandates of the organization's lawyers. In some areas where patients or professionals are under ethical duress, the law is as much in need of direction as it is able to provide it. The specific relation of organization ethics to compliance should not be one of subordination—a point we address further in Chapter 10. For all these reasons, we believe location of the organization ethics program in the legal department will lead to its marginalization and quash any hope of its being a positive force for the HCO, its patients, professionals, managers, and its community.

Professional staff

Should the organization ethics program, like many clinical ethics programs, be controlled by the professional staff of an organization? Doctors, nurses, and other healthcare professionals have a strong professional identity articulated and maintained by their professional codes, which should assure their independence from the protective impulses of the CEO or organizational attorney. They have an avowed obligation to protect the interests of the primary stakeholder in a HCO, the patient. Since the mission and ethical climate that is developed and maintained by the organization ethics program should reflect this same obligation as one of its primary goals, is this not an ideal fit for the organization ethics program? Again, we believe not.

Although patient care will always be at the core of any HCO, it is not the only area for valid claims of ethical consideration. There are major obligations to employees, to payers for health care, to regulators and accreditors, to contractual partners, to the patient community, and society in general. Adequate representation of these interests by the organization ethics program is necessary, and consideration of these issues by healthcare professionals alone would be understandably suspect.

Ideal location

Given these shortcomings, it is our strong recommendation that the organization ethics program should be administratively located as an advisor to (and possibly an occasional decision maker for) the governing board. It should have authority to conduct its activities without being structurally subordinated to the administration, legal department, or professional areas of the HCO. Figure 9.1 identifies a common healthcare organization structure and how an organization ethics program should fit into this structure.

The advantages to both the HCO and the organization ethics program itself in locating the program at the board level are obvious. Prestige and authority for the program are crucial if it is to succeed, and prestige and authority are guaranteed for board-level activities. Decisions concerning adequate funding for the required work should be associated with little or no controversy, and allocation of the necessary funds will be automatic with board support. When the organization ethics program has strong support from the board, consultation with the program by all aspects of the HCO should rapidly become accepted and routine, acceptance and understanding of the role of the organization ethics program should be enhanced throughout the organization, and, most importantly, there should be no undue influence by any particular department of the organization. Locating the organization ethics program at the board level will allow it to do its work in relative harmony and understanding in all areas of the HCO,

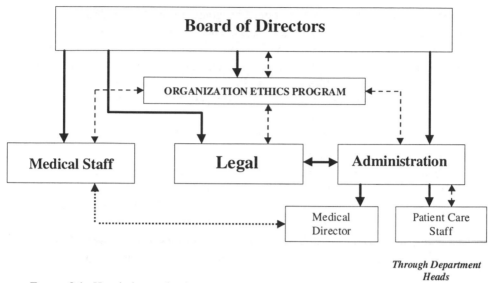

FIGURE 9.1. Hospital organization structure.

including administration, professional staff, and the legal department. Any other location for the program will make its task more difficult and likely delay or impede its development.

This does not mean that an organization ethics program, without a specific mandate and direct authority from the governing board, should be able to promulgate directives, guidelines, or policies, which are antagonistic to the position of the senior administration, professional staff, patients, or legal advisors. It also does not mean that an organization ethics program should function without input and discussion from each of these important stakeholders. Organization ethics program membership should include representatives from each of these areas assuring representation of particular viewpoints. It does mean, however, that the organization ethics program will always be able to look at the organization as a whole and consider how particular actions or decisions promote or detract from the goal of developing a consistent positive ethical climate.

WILL PATIENT CARE ETHICS ACTIVITIES BE ADDRESSED BY THE ORGANIZATION ETHICS PROGRAM?

There are well integrated, fully functioning clinical or patient care ethics committees, often referred to as institutional ethics committees (IECs), of relatively long standing in most HCOs. Should the accepted activities of this committee become a part of the organization ethics program? From the standpoint of the patient care ethics committee, the answer is not necessarily yes. The focus of IECs is often on particular patient dilemmas. Some committee members might fear that the committee's mandate will be diluted or that its focus will become fuzzy if it is folded into a committee with a different scope. Further, many members of patient care ethics committees are not ready for such a change. These members have fought a battle for appropriate recognition of the patient care ethics activities and do not wish to see the advances they have made subordinated to the whims of a more globally focused committee or program.

Others look at this issue differently. Paul Schyve, a senior official of the JCAHO,* has suggested that the most efficient and effective way for an HCO to fulfill its requirements for "organization ethics" under the JCAHO standards would be to expand the role of the institutional patient care ethics committee. On this model, the now expanded ethics committees would be given responsibility for overseeing the development of an ethical framework for the business and managerial operation of the HCO.

The suggestion that the patient care ethics committee be expanded in both membership and responsibility to include professional and managerial considerations is one which deserves full consideration; we will discuss this issue more fully later in this chapter. One alternative to this is to disband the present IECs and constitute an organization ethics program that has responsibility for patient care ethical issues along with ethical issues from other areas of the HCO. These alternatives to some extent constitute a distinction without a difference, at least in terms of process. Whichever alternative is chosen, the responsibilities for ethical consideration throughout the organization are expanded and the membership broadened to meet those responsibilities. The positive effect on the organization should be the same.

HOW AND TO WHAT EXTENT WILL PROFESSIONAL ETHICS ISSUES BE ADDRESSED BY AN ORGANIZATION ETHICS PROGRAM?

In Chapter 5 we discussed the relationship between the traditional ethical stance of doctors and nurses and the objectives of the organization ethics program. Often these perspectives will be complementary. We do not consider organization ethics a replacement for professional ethics, and suggest that an effective organization ethics program needs to protect and foster the professional ethics of

---

*Schyve suggested in a talk given to Virginia Bioethics Network members in October 1995 in Charlottesville, Virginia, that ethics committee members are most qualified to take the lead in formulating and implementing organization ethics programs.

professionals. In discussing the relation between stakeholder theory and organization ethics in Chapter 4, we emphasized the importance of reciprocity in the relations between the HCO and its stakeholders or stakeholder groups in exemplary organizations. Reciprocal responsibility is well illustrated in the relation between the HCO and the professionals who deliver care.

Because the primary activity of the HCO as well as its reputation depends on the professionals, it is necessary for the professional ethics perspective to be an integral part of the organization ethics program. With the help of the clinical staffs, this program will need to develop and maintain a consistent positive support of professional obligations within the HCO where the patient is being treated. On the other side, professional groups within HCOs represent specific standards of practice and retain various prerogatives of access to practice, discipline, task allocation and self regulation, and the HCO, as well as the public in general, expects the actions of professionals to conform to those standards. The close association of these two perspectives and the status and authority of the organization ethics program within the HCO suggest that the program should be the site for professional ethics issues to be discussed and resolved should the professional standards not be met, or should the retained prerogatives not be exercised responsibly.

The organization ethics program might equally well serve as the site for discussion of decisions, structures, strategies, policies, or contracts that members of professional groups judge to be threats to their ethical practice. Organization ethics committee members must understand that consideration of obligations articulated by professional organizations will be an important part of the discussion of professional ethics issues. The professional obligations articulated by specific professional codes set the parameters within which the healthcare professional expects to operate while working within the HCO. This mutual expectation and reciprocal responsibility and respect is a good example of the relationship which an HCO might aspire to have with all its stakeholders, and which organization ethics, as we understand it, hopes to facilitate.

In practical terms ethical guidelines for professionals within an HCO will be determined via a two-tiered system. The basic ethical tenets to which all in the profession should adhere is determined in the traditional manner, via longstanding, slowly changing codes maintained by independent professional organizations. The second tier, the ethical basis for most everyday decisions within the HCO, will be articulated and maintained via the HCO itself, with the organization ethics program exercising primary responsibility for maintaining necessary guidelines or codes for professional behavior within the particular HCO. It may be necessary in some HCOs to have a standing subcommittee of the organization ethics program to oversee these crucial activities and to deal with conflicts of commitment that may arise between mandates of the HCO and perceived external professional requirements.

SHOULD AN ORGANIZATION ETHICS PROGRAM
BE ADVISORY ONLY, OR SHOULD IT HAVE LIMITED
(OR EXTENDED) DECISION-MAKING AUTHORITY?

So far in this chapter we have recommended designating knowledgeable and committed individuals from the most critical areas of the HCO to devote time to the organization ethics program. We have recommended that it be located at the level of the board of directors, and have given it responsibility for the morale, reputation, and eventually the competitive advantage of the HCO. Surely it would be paradoxical to demand that it be granted respect, visibility, and authority, and yet to deny it the capacity to make decisions. Nonetheless, we believe that in order to maintain its moral authority, the organization ethics program should make as few decisions as possible.

Behind this paradox lies a lively debate about the proper role of ethics in institutions. On the one hand is the image of the ethics committee as a site of technical expertise, commanding a field of expert knowledge, problem-solving skills, experience, and technique, called upon to solve ethical problems as a neurologist might be called in to resolve a particular kind of medical problem. An alternative model sees the role of ethics in an institution as facilitating communication, clarifying moral positions, and arranging a safe moral space within which differences can be aired, understood, and in some (if not all) cases resolved. Both models have something to contribute to clinical ethics, and even those of us who see the task of ethics as communication and consensus building acknowledge that a considerable knowledge and skill base is required. But the pragmatic approach to clinical ethics described in Chapter 3, like the organization ethics program this book recommends, views expertise and experience as useful tools for achieving a procedural consensus rather than guarantors of the "right" answer. Our approach to organization ethics derives the moral authority of the program from this role in the institution (Casarett, Frona & Lantos, 1998).

As we emphasized above, in order to gain and retain respect in the HCO, an organization ethics program must be perceived at all levels of the HCO as representative, unbiased, independent, and with no specific agenda beyond the articulation and maintenance of the mission and the enhancement of a positive ethical climate in the HCO. Our conception of the organization ethics program as properly facilitating and mediating change, rather than legislating it, requires that it make as few specific decisions as possible. Thus we suggest that the organization ethics program have mainly an advisory function, with the actual decision-making authority being maintained in the traditional areas of the HCO. Administrative and overall policy decisions should continue to be made by the governing board and administration; medical decisions by patients, families, and healthcare professionals. Broader social and legal decisions affecting on the HCO will continue to be made by the community via laws and community mores.

An organization ethics program might be more than an advisory body in the area of compliance activities as dictated by federal law and discussed in Chapter 10. Under certain well-defined, specific circumstances it may be advisable for the program to have decision-making authority. If the organization ethics program has some responsibility for compliance activities within the HCO, it will be necessary by law and regulation for some decisions to be made by the organization ethics program members. For instance, the guidelines concerning the features of an adequate compliance program include requirements that the person or group responsible for compliance activities accept responsibility for certain educational and auditing activities that may require decision-making authority.

This authority, although necessary in this limited area, needs to be well defined by policies based on applicable laws and regulations, and should always be subject to review by the governing board or another department designated by the board. With this exception, the organization ethics program should begin and remain as primarily an advisory function, but one that has the responsibility and full authority to address any issue that may have an impact on the ethical climate of the organization.

WHAT AUTHORITY DOES AN ORGANIZATION ETHICS PROGRAM HAVE TO INFLUENCE DECISIONS CONCERNING CONTRACTUAL AND OTHER RELATIONSHIPS TO ENTITIES THAT DO NOT ADHERE TO THE SAME ETHICAL STANCE?

What can the HCO do to protect itself, its constituencies, and the patients it serves, from external demands that threaten its ethical stance? This question is at the heart of the challenge to HCOs in the current tumultuous, precarious, and competitive environment. It is the question that prompted the authors to write this book. The organization ethics process, as we have developed it throughout this book, is in our view the best hope for an answer. Although MCO contracts may be the most widely publicized contracts that raise this question today, the problem of relationships to entities with different ethical expectations is one which can arise in relationship with any individual stakeholder or stakeholder group.

Activities of HCOs are defined by contracts and relationships with both internal and external stakeholders. As agents outside the HCO, external stakeholders are not under its direct control. Attempting to maintain an HCO's core values and positive ethical climate in dealings with these external entities may, at times, be problematic. For example, an HCO may support ethical standards that articulate as a primary tenet the mandate for full and honest disclosure of actual and potential conflicts of interest or commitment that could conceivably have an effect on decisions concerning the care of particular patients. If this HCO has a contract with a managed care organization that does not adhere to the same ethical standard, the HCO may find its capacity to meet this expectation called into question. The HCO will quickly discover that it is judged on the basis of a contract that overrides one of its basic ethical tenets rather than on its stated values. Other examples abound of the actual ethical performance of an HCO being undermined by contractual obligations that are antagonistic to the stated ethical standards of the HCO.

Since agents external to the HCO are not under its control, it may not always realistically be possible to determine the conditions of all its contractual relations. Remember, however, that the positive or negative value of an organization's ethical climate is not entirely dependent upon the content of the expectations, but is at least partially a function of whether or not the organization is seen to be living up to those expectations, whatever the content may be. Explicit discussion with contractual partners concerning the ethical issues implicit in the contractual relationship may not immediately be able to improve the contract. But by increasing the understanding of the affected stakeholders, the HCO may be able to salvage institutional morale by informing constituents' expectations. At this moment in history HCOs can not necessarily change circumstances at will. But an institution can always choose to deal openly, honestly, and explicitly with its various stakeholder groups. People who know what is going on are less likely to be angry, fearful, disappointed, or surprised.

Relations with external stakeholders is the most difficult challenge institutions face if truly committed to their ethical standards, for a HCO cannot be a truly ethical entity without assuming responsibility for extending the mandates of its mission to all activities the HCO is involved in, including contractual relationships outside the organization. The HCO has no authority to impose its core values on other individuals or organizations in any activities beyond their relationships with the HCO, but it can expect that its ethical standards be a basic foundation of any contract or relationship which the HCO has with another person or organization. Otherwise the HCO cannot achieve a positive ethical climate within the organization no matter what its avowed standards are. An organization ethics program must be involved in helping the HCO assure that its mission and core values will be maintained in all of its contractual relationships. Although this will be a major undertaking, it is one without which the activities and goals of the organization ethics program can have little meaning.

Relationships with persons and institutions outside the HCO are commonly defined by contracts of varying lengths. The institution of an organization ethics program in a given HCO may not coincide with the beginning or renewal of all these contracts, so consideration needs to be given to how the contractual obligations of the HCO, which may not correspond to the newly articulated goal of developing a positive ethical climate consistent with its mission, will be addressed by the HCO. The organization ethics program needs to consider this issue and make recommendations to the administration and the governing board concerning those contracts that do not comply to one or more core tenets of the statements defining the ethical standards. If there is a legal or compliance problem, it must be addressed immediately and, with the help of the HCO's legal department, the contracts revised as necessary.

Whatever the length of the contract, all entities with a contractual relationship with the HCO should be informed of the core values that frame the HCO's decision making, and informed that these values must be adhered to in any future contract negotiations or renewals. This will alert an HCO's contractual partners that the HCO is serious about its ethical stance and that its mission statement defines the parameters of any relationship it has. Although this may present problems for some contractual partners of the HCO, it should also be reassuring to them, since it is a concrete demonstration of the commitment of a HCO to defining itself as an ethical entity. The trust engendered may ultimately be beneficial to the HCO and its contractual partners. An organization ethics program should oversee this process with input from all affected areas of the HCO and with open communication with its contractual partners.

HOW WILL THE ORGANIZATION ETHICS PROGRAM BE STRUCTURED?

The issues and activities of the organization ethics program were defined in the previous chapter and discussed here, so the major remaining practical question is how the organization ethics program should be structured. Of course, different institutions will have different needs and will have to accommodate their programs to the resources they have available. In this section we will present one model of how to structure an organization ethics program. This may serve as a useful provisional standard against which to evaluate a program in the process of development by a HCO.

We have given reasons why we believe that the organization ethics program should be located administratively as a function of the governing board, but the question remains of how to organize the organization ethics program to enable it to fulfill its functions in an efficient and appropriate manner. The patient care ethics committee might be the host locus for the development of the organization ethics program, and there are reasons, some of which we discuss in chapter 10, why this may be a good place to start. If this is to be considered, and we believe it should be, several issues need to be addressed.

Traditionally, patient care ethics committees or IECs have had a limited mission, often explicitly noted as such in their mission statements or operating bylaws. Most patient care ethics committees, as we noted in Chapter 3, support certain major activities, including the development and presentation of educational programs related to ethical issues, review of institutional policies that have a direct impact on the ethics of the care of individual patients, and consultation for staff, patients, and others concerning perceived ethical problems related to a specific patient's care. In fact, expanding the role of presently constituted patient care ethics committees to include broader institutional ethics issues has received little practical consideration, either by most patient care committee members or from most organization ethics development committees. There are legitimate reasons for this lack of interest by patient care ethics committees, including at least the following:

1. A preoccupation with individual patient and professional issues
2. A lack of appropriate knowledge and/or training of patient care ethics committee members
3. A requirement for expansion of education and policy development activities into new areas
4. Difficulty in defining appropriate ethical parameters for decision making in the business and management arenas, and to some degree in professional areas
5. Difficulty in understanding and addressing federal compliance and sentencing guidelines
6. A reluctance to become involved in the more allegedly "sleazy" aspects of health care—those aspects surrounding the appropriate acquisition and spending of money and responding to complicated regulations

These are substantive and important objections to the expansion of the role of the patient care ethics committee and HCOs should consider them when deciding how to proceed with the development of their organization ethics program. These objections do not, however, necessarily preclude changing the direction of and adding to the accepted focus of the work of the patient care ethics committee and using it as the base for building the organization ethics program (Spencer, 1997a, p. 373).

There are a number of good reasons why an HCO should add the organization ethics program activities to the functions of an expanded patient care ethics committee. They include:

1. Who better? It is true that IECs or patient care ethics committees have little or no experience as yet with the ethics issues of business and management, compliance issues, or professional ethics issues, but ethical consideration and discussion is a function of the patient care ethics committee now. Consideration and discussion focusing on organizational ethics issues will require enhancement of the knowledge of present members of the patient care ethics committee and the addition of new members with the requisite knowledge. However, the methods for consideration of the organizational ethics issues should not change and present committee members are already familiar with these methods.

2. Since the role and function of an organization ethics program is new to the institution, any committee, whether established completely of new members or reconstituted and supplemented from an extant ethics committee, will require reorientation and additional education.
3. The patient care ethics committee is already in place. In most HCOs it is a recognized source for education and advice on ethics issues. Asking this committee to expand and do the same type of work in different arenas seems efficient and logical.
4. The work required to develop the organizational code of ethics mandated by the JCAHO and the policies supporting this code is familiar to most ethics committees, since most have had experience with the analysis and development of guidelines and policies pertaining to ethical issues and have a working knowledge of other codes of ethics. The compliance and professional arenas are more problematic, but these would be new activities for any committee and, with appropriate consultation and help, they should be able to be addressed by an expanded patient care ethics committee as well as by any other structure.

To choose the IEC as the base for developing the organization ethics program is in effect to restructure and rededicate that committee. All of the previously mentioned issues affecting the development and work of the organization ethics program need to be considered in this context and decisions made concerning the required expansion of mission and personnel. The existing patient care ethics committee will have to expand its membership to fulfill JCAHO requirements concerning the business and financial operations of the HCO. How to adequately address compliance issues, and what the reciprocal responsibilities are between the professional staff and the HCO must be added to the task of maintaining appropriate attention to ethical issues in patient care.

A realistic plan for the organization and function of the organization ethics committee is encompassed in the following four recommendations. (See Figure 9.2 for a schematic representation of the structure and function of an organization ethics committee.)

Recommendation I: Prior to taking on the new responsibility, the IEC should either expand to include members from all-important departments of the HCO or reorganize in a manner recommended by the organization ethics development team. Whatever route for change is chosen, inclusion of representatives from the administration, board of directors, business office, billing office, internal (and possibly external) professional groups, and legal or risk-management representatives knowledgeable about compliance issues, as well as patient care representatives is mandatory. It must also expand to include healthcare professionals interested in and qualified to develop the professional ethics aspect of the organization ethics program. Many of the healthcare professionals already members of the patient care ethics committee may be willing and able to undertake this task but attention must

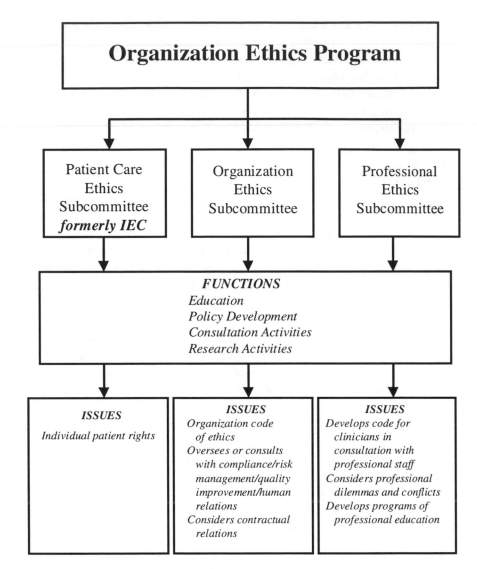

FIGURE 9.2. Structure and function of an organization ethics program.

be given to others affected by this work: others such as the organized medical staff, the administrative nursing staff, and possibly outsiders such as representatives from local professional organizations. The representatives who will be responsible for the compliance efforts are relatively well spelled out in federal guidelines and include legal and administrative representative. The major difference for this function is that it now will have the full organization ethics program as a clearinghouse for its final recommendations and activities except where specifically mandated differently by federal law or regulation.

Recommendation II: The reformulated larger committee should be divided into four subcommittees: the patient care subcommittee which will continue the direct patient care focused activities of the former IEC; the management and organization ethics subcommittee which will be responsible for the development of an appropriate organizational code of ethics, as well as for development of policies and of the mechanisms needed to assure that the code is effective and that the policies are appropriate; the professional ethics subcommittee, which will address professional obligations and conflicts within the HCO as outlined above; and the corporate compliance subcommittee, which will oversee all functions related to federal law and regulations mandated by the federal government. (Spencer, 1997a, p. 374)

The membership of the patient care subcommittee will remain mainly clinical, but with the addition of one or more representatives from each of the three other subcommittees. The management and organizational ethics subcommittee will consist mainly of representatives from the business and managerial departments of the HCO with one or more representatives from each of the other subcommittees. The professional ethics subcommittee will consist of members from actively practicing healthcare professionals within the HCO, one or more representatives from the organized medical staff and the administrative nursing staff, and representatives from professional organizations outside the HCO as needed and as dictated by the circumstances, plus one or more members from each of the other subcommittees. The corporate compliance subcommittee will consist of representatives from the administration, legal department, and risk management, plus one or more representatives from each of the other subcommittees.

Recommendation III: The organization ethics committee will continue to be advisory only (with the possible exception mentioned in relation to the requirements of the compliance subcommittee) with the ultimate responsibility for adoption and institution of codes, policies, guidelines, and particular actions residing with the governing Board of the HCO. (Spencer, 1997a, p. 374)

Recommendation IV: The entire organization ethics committee will make all recommendations to the Board after full consideration and discussion of each subcommittee's work. For some larger HCOs this may be too cumbersome and may need to be modified to allow each subcommittee to issue its own reports and recommendations directly to the board. However, any recommendation which directly affects the ethical standards or the ethical climate should emanate from the full committee or from all of the combined subcommittees acting in concert. (p. 375)

The initial lack of expertise of the patient care ethics committee members in business and management, professional, and compliance areas can be overcome by the input from new members with expertise in these areas. On the whole we consider the advantages of the newly expanded ethics committee remaining the site within the HCO for ethical discussion and consensus building to outweigh the disadvantages.

CONCLUSION

Considerable effort is required to start and continue a comprehensive organization ethics program. There are numerous ways for this program to reach the goal of developing and supporting a meaningful positive ethical climate for the HCO. In this chapter we have discussed processes to be considered when undertaking this task and have made a number of suggestions that should be helpful to those responsible for an HCO's organization ethics program.

10

Compliance, Risk-Management, and Quality-Improvement Programs

The public's negative perceptions of the healthcare system have led to calls for regulation and will likely lead to further, possibly expensive changes. These in turn will increase the need for HCOs to develop mechanisms to protect their position in the marketplace. Programs addressing compliance, risk management, and continuous quality improvement are already part of the HCO's administrative structure or soon will be. If these programs are seen as mechanisms that help protect or strengthen the HCO in the market, then these programs and their influence in the HCO will certainly grow.

At first glance, these three activities may appear to either duplicate the healthcare organization ethics program or offer a framework that can easily be expanded to encompass the goals of such a program. In this chapter we argue otherwise. To make this argument we will first consider the role in the current HCO structure of these three programs. We will then consider whether one or more of these programs should be expanded to include the organization ethics program.

Our view is that although corporate compliance programs, risk-management programs, and continuous quality-improvement programs fulfill other important goals of the HCO, they are not sufficient to ensure the sound ethical climate of a HCO. The converse is not true. An effective healthcare organization ethics program can support the goals and activities surrounding each of the three.

CORPORATE COMPLIANCE

Seeking to correct what was perceived by many critics as unevenly applied justice, Congress passed the Sentencing Reform Act of 1984 (Title II of the Comprehensive Crime Control Act of 1984). The Sentencing Reform Act established the United States Sentencing Commission, an independent agency in the judicial branch composed of seven voting and two nonvoting ex officio members. The commission's purpose is to establish sentencing policies and practices for the federal criminal justice system that will assure the ends of justice by promulgating detailed guidelines prescribing the appropriate sentences for offenders convicted of federal crimes (Federal Sentencing Guidelines, 1995b). The result of the commission's work is the Federal Sentencing Guidelines.

These guidelines distinguish different levels of criminal activity and specify the appropriate restitution and punishment associated with that activity. The sentencing court must elect a sentence from within the guideline range, and it may not depart from a guideline-specified sentence unless a particular case presents atypical features. The court must specify the reasons for any departure from these guidelines (p. 1). Failure to follow the sentencing guidelines may result in an appeal by either the defendant or the government (Dalton, Metzger & Hill, 1994).

In 1991 an extension of the guidelines applied them to organizations found guilty of violating federal law (Federal Sentencing Guidelines, 1995a). The guidelines state that an "organization" means "a person other than an individual." "Persons" under this definition include: corporations, partnerships, associations, joint stock companies, unions, trusts, pension funds, unincorporated organizations, governments and their political subdivisions, and nonprofit organizations (p. 2). Healthcare organizations, whether nonprofit or for-profit, incorporated or unincorporated, are included under this definition.

Chapter 8 of the Federal Sentencing Guidelines addresses guidelines and policy statements when the convicted defendant is an organization. According to Chapter 8's introductory commentary, even though individual agents are responsible for their own criminal conduct, organizations are additionally vicariously liable for offenses committed by their agents, and as such can be held culpable for the individual's actions (p. 1). Organizations may therefore be responsible for any financial restitution or punishment associated with an individual's criminal behavior while acting as an agent or employee of the organization. The range of fines or other punishments for the organization is based on the seriousness of the offense and the culpability of the organization.

The guidelines, however, offer potential mitigation of organization culpability by tying culpability to steps taken by the organization, before the offense occurs, to prevent and detect criminal conduct, the level and extent of involvement in or tolerance of the offense by certain personnel, and the organization's actions after an offense has been committed (p. 1). The commission recognizes that an organization cannot control every action taken by every individual associated with the organization. But organizations can try to promote a climate in which it is unacceptable to break the law. Organizations can do this through effective programs to prevent and detect violations of the law (p. 5). Evidence that efforts in this direction have been made reduces the level of culpability and thus the cost to the organization.

These programs, called corporate compliance programs, are so important that organization attorneys who do not review compliance within their organization may be considered guilty of "recklessness" (Dalton, Metzger & Hill, 1994, p. 332). If such a program is in place, then organization culpability is reduced, as are the fines or punishment the organization may otherwise receive. Richard L. Clarke, president and CEO of the Healthcare Financial Management Association, states that corporate compliance is not optional. Professionals who fail to install a comprehensive corporate compliance plan, or who neglect current regulations, are gambling with their professional and personal futures, as well as with the future of the organization of which they are members. (Healthcare Financial Management Association Press Release, 1997). Department of Justice (DOJ) and Office of Inspector General (OIG) officials have stated that if an organization has in place a visible and effective compliance program, fines may be mitigated (Healthcare Financial Management Association Express News, 1997). Since there is no guaranteed protection against individual wrongdoing in any organization, organizations, including HCOs, have a powerful motive to establish visible corporate compliance programs.

Chapter 8 of the Federal Sentencing Guidelines states what the Sentencing Commission considers the hallmarks of an effective compliance program:

1. The organization must have established compliance standards and procedures to be followed by its employees and other agents that are reasonably capable of reducing the prospect of criminal conduct.
2. Specific individual(s) within high-level personnel of the organization must have been assigned overall responsibility to oversee compliance with such standards and procedures.
3. The organization must have used due care not to delegate substantial discretionary authority to individuals whom the organization knew, or should have known through the exercise of due diligence, had a propensity to engage in illegal activities.
4. The organization must have taken steps to communicate effectively its standards and procedures to all employees and other agents, e.g., by requiring participation in training programs or by disseminating publications that explain in a practical manner what is required.
5. The organization must have taken reasonable steps to achieve compliance with its standards, e.g., by utilizing monitoring and auditing systems rea-

sonably designed to detect criminal conduct by its employees and other agents and by having in place and publicizing a reporting system whereby employees and other agents could report criminal conduct by others within the organization without fear of retribution.

6. The standards must have been consistently enforced through appropriate disciplinary mechanisms, including, as appropriate, discipline of individuals responsible for the failure to detect an offense. Adequate discipline of individuals responsible for an offense is a necessary component of enforcement; however, the form of discipline that will be appropriate will be case specific.

7. After an offense has been detected, the organization must have taken all reasonable steps to respond appropriately to the offense and to prevent further similar offenses including any necessary modifications to its program to prevent and detect violations of law. (Federal Sentencing Guidelines, 1995)

To the question of what DOJ officials will deem effective, the Federal Sentencing Guidelines offer some suggestions:

1. Make corporate compliance the responsibility of a high level administrator;
2. Implement appropriate (independent or not) audit procedures to detect fraud or other abuses;
3 Sponsor training programs for its employees that include accountability issues;
4. Ensure that penalties for wrong-doing are highly publicized throughout the organization;
5. Establish a hot-line for employees to report wrong-doing without fear of reprisals;
6. Document these activities and make them accessible to all employees. (Federal Sentencing Guidelines, 1995)

COMPLIANCE AND ITS RELATIONSHIP TO THE GOALS OF HEALTHCARE ORGANIZATION ETHICS PROGRAM

The main goal of a corporate compliance program from the DOJ perspective is to promote the organization's compliance with the law. The DOJ in its report, *Health Care Fraud Report Fiscal Years 1995–1996* (U.S. Department of Justice, 1999), calls healthcare fraud the "Crisis of the Nineties" (p. 3). The number of healthcare fraud investigations by the Federal Bureau of Investigation (which works closely with the DOJ) increased from 657 in fiscal year 1992 to 2,200 in fiscal year 1996 (p. 3). These investigations have resulted in an increased number of guilty pleas and guilty verdicts. The DOJ states in its report that it has been and intends to continue to be aggressive in identifying and punishing healthcare fraud—in billing, unbundling, kickbacks, and misrepresentations—by "individual physicians as well as multi-state publicly traded companies, medical equipment dealers, ambulance companies, and laboratories as well as the hospitals, nursing homes, and home health agencies they service" (p. 4). The aggressive campaign waged against what the DOJ calls "this scourge against the integrity of our nation's healthcare system" (p. 3) has had the effect of making healthcare executives take particular note of one avenue of avoidance of possible punishment for wrongdoing—a corporate compliance program. HCO corporate compliance programs, to date, have a focused and specific function related to illegal activities—to prevent them and avoid DOJ attention or, in a worst-case scenario, mitigate the punishment for wrongdoing. With this preoccupation, current HCO corporate compliance programs neither have the time nor the interest in providing mechanisms that are capable of promoting and enhancing a positive ethical climate within the HCO beyond ensuring compliance with the law.

Could an expanded compliance program encompass the goals of the healthcare organization ethics program? An HCO may decide to expand its compliance activities so that the compliance program oversees the development and implementation of policies, procedures, reporting functions, and other accrediting requirements the HCO must fulfill to maintain JCAHO (or other) accreditation. This would technically fulfill accreditation requirements. But is this wise if the organization is serious about the goals of an organization ethics program?

In a recent study Gary R. Weaver and Linda K. Treviño identify and explore the effects of two types of ethics programs on corporate behavior (Weaver & Treviño, 1999). Weaver and Treviño call the first type of ethics program "compliance" oriented and the second type of ethics program "values" oriented. Compliance-oriented ethics programs emphasize rules, monitor employee behavior, and discipline misconduct. Values-oriented programs emphasize support for employees' ethical aspirations and the development of shared values (p. 3).

Weaver and Treviño argue that both types of programs seek to "bring some degree of order and predictability to employee behavior" (p. 4) and that the two orientations are not mutually exclusive. For example, a values-oriented ethics program could exist with rules, accountability, and disciplinary mechanisms (p. 6). But according to Weaver and Treviño, their studies of both types of programs indicate that, all things being equal, "a focus on monitoring and discipline in an ethics program is more likely to engender a contractual employee attitude toward the organization, rather than a perception of organizational support and trust, or increased salience for one ethical obligation as an organizational member" (p. 2). We understand a "contractual employee attitude" to mean an attitude where shared values between the organization and employee are irrelevant—the employee is to perform some function for which that employee is paid and that employee is monitored to ensure that function is performed. But Weaver and

Treviño indicate that according to their data, a focus on monitoring implies distrust of employees, and this may encourage a response to the ethics program which is calculated and self-interested. This response is hardly likely to encourage organizational commitment or communication (p. 13).

Communication, of course, is at the heart of an effective compliance program. Thus, it seems that there is a contradiction. Communication is needed for an effective compliance program, but Weaver and Treviño supply data suggesting that a compliance program without a value-orientation encourages noncommunication: "A values-orientation, in particular, appears to add distinctive and desirable outcomes that cannot be achieved by a perceived focus on behavioral compliance. Moreover, a values-orientation appears important to fully realizing the potential benefits of compliance activities such as reporting misconduct" (p.18). Since an organization ethics program is a values-based program—it appears that it may be more effective to subsume the goals of the compliance program to the goals of the organization ethics program than the converse. An organization can accomplish compliance within the context of an organization ethics program, but an organization may not be able to support the values it says it endorses within the context of a compliance program.

RISK MANAGEMENT

Risk management is one of the specialties within the field of management. It has two aspects, a managerial focus and a decisional aspect. One definition of risk management, which combines these two aspects, is the process of making and carrying out decisions that will minimize the adverse effects of accidental losses upon an organization (Neilson, 1998). Implicit in this definition is the idea that risk management is concerned with the identification, evaluation, and prevention of accidental losses (including losses from unforeseen lawsuits) that may result in financial loss to the organization, and may prevent the organization from fulfilling its mission.

Traditionally, the risk manager in an HCO has been concerned with this narrow view of risk management. Areas which have been identified as exposing the HCO to risk include workers' compensation for occupational illness and employee injuries, patient and visitor injuries, transportation accidents, exposures to hazardous waste, embezzlement, fraud in third-party reimbursement, breaches of contract, and defamation charges. However, the largest single issue that has historically occupied the attention of risk managers within an HCO is providing protection against medical malpractice for its professional medical staff (Carson, Carson & Roe, 1995).

The risk manager employs three strategies to protect an HCO. These strategies, sometimes called control functions, include risk prevention, risk avoidance, and risk shifting (Carson, Carson & Roe, 1995, pp. 351–353). The risk manager may implement educational programs to alert employees to workplace hazards (risk prevention), the HCO may drop certain healthcare services because of their potential for lawsuits (risk avoidance), or the HCO may decide to transfer the responsibility of offering certain healthcare services to another organization or group (risk shifting). Thus, the traditional approach of risk management in HCOs has been to prevent, minimize, or recover losses to the HCO.

This role of risk management in HCOs is changing, however. HCOs must pay ever more attention to the characteristics of the market in order to survive (Mulligan, Shapiro & Walrod, 1996). Previously, areas of risk management answered questions of how to provide certain healthcare services at the lowest risk exposure consistent with the organization's mission. However, the growth of managed care has caused significant changes in contractual relationships between the HCO and payers. These changing contractual relationships will inevitably enhance the role of risk management within the HCO as risk managers seek not only to limit risk exposure within the HCO, but also to control the positive risk-reward tradeoff that is represented in such contractual arrangements as capitation agreements. Today, risk management is (or should be) an integral part of the strategic planning process undertaken by HCO leadership. This is because the level and type of risk borne by the HCO, and the resulting contractual relationships the HCO forms with other providers, will in large part determine the financial viability of the HCO. In other words, the mandate of the risk management team is not only to help the HCO recover from accidental or unplanned losses, but also to gain from the organization's exposure to certain kinds of risk. Thus, the role of risk management in HCOs has moved beyond those considerations of risk associated with liability losses and is now seen (or should be seen) as a core activity of the HCO. Inevitably, the responsibility and influence of risk management within the HCO will grow as its activities broaden, and this expanded responsibility will touch upon the ethics of the HCO.

Consider, for instance, two types of risk any HCO must consider as examples of how decisions made by the risk manager may impact clinical, professional, and business ethics within the HCO. They are:

1   Clinical operating risk—the risk variations in the costs incurred by a payer, a professional, or provider in providing healthcare services; and

2   Event risk—the risk associated with fluctuating demand for health care in the population served by the HCO. (Mulligan, Shapiro & Walrod, p. 96)

Managing clinical operating risk means managing two components: treatment-management risk and cost-management risk. The risk associated with treatment management can arise from the doctor's choice between alternative treatments or because different patients respond in different ways to the same treatment. Cost-management risk is driven by variations in the cost of the elements of care, including the behavior of those contractually linked to the HCO who are providing services (p. 98).

Risk management had little concern with either treatment-management risk or cost-management risk in a fee-for-service world. There was no need to be concerned with variations when the expenses associated with these variations would be covered by third-party payers. In a capitated world, however, risk managers are not only interested in controlling clinical operating risk by reviewing and standardizing treatment protocols, but may consider as well strategies of influencing treatment choices of professionals through the use of various incentives. As well documented in the literature (Clancy, 1995; Emanuel, 1995; Holleman, Edwards & Matson, 1994; Iglehart, 1994) such incentives may conflict directly with professional mandates assuring a conflict of interest by providing the professional with incentives to undertreat.

Event risk management has to do with forecasting and managing those events that occur outside the HCO but which have the potential to affect the HCO. For instance, what is the patient population served? Is that population changing? What kind of cost-service variation is implied through this change? What is the size and mix of the pool of patients served? What is the likelihood of new regulations forcing the HCO to change the way it operates? What decisions should the HCO make to ensure that it gains through these changes?

Consider, for instance, a strategy of event risk management called risk unbundling, which is another form of risk shifting. Risk unbundling occurs when the HCO retains a small premium and passes the risk of providing a certain type of care to a different party. Risk unbundling can occur through the use of capitation agreements, or through the use of a gatekeeper. These strategies are intended to modify behavior, and they have the same effect as that intended with withholds or bonuses. They set up a conflict of interest that, if acted upon, may profoundly affect either physician or administrative behavior, and which therefore may directly affect ethical decisions made within the HCO.

The way in which an HCO reacts to changes in the market, or the way it seeks to affect the market, will affect not only the entire HCO, but also the community the HCO serves. These strategic decisions will certainly affect the structure of an HCO, and they have the potential to change its very mission. Because of this potential, these decisions should be made within the context of the core values of the healthcare organization. It is these values that are protected and enhanced by a healthcare organization ethics program.

The function and obligation of HCO risk management is to protect the organization and help position it strategically to assume appropriate risk and to gain through avoidance of unnecessary risk. While the risk manager may have to be aware of and address compliance issues, the risk manager's goal is to protect the organization financially while simultaneously seeking ways to save costs and increase opportunities. Inevitably, there will be conflicts between what risk management legitimately perceives as being an appropriate risk profile for the whole organization, and the particular values of its various individual stakeholders—its patients, professionals, and community.

Relationship of risk management to organization ethics

There is little doubt that the role of risk management in HCOs has grown and will continue to grow. Since appropriate risk assumption may very well determine overall organization viability, decisions taken by risk managers will inevitably be taken within the context of the organization core strategies. These decisions are and should be seen as decisions that try to ensure organizational survival and financial stability. Risk management may use incentives that seek to influence behavior and treatment guidelines to achieve organization goals. As sophisticated risk-management strategies develop, they may clash with the principles and values driving clinical, professional, and business ethics within HCOs, and this potential for conflict will increase as the competitive pressures in the market continue and the role of risk management increases. Clearly, then, organization ethics processes cannot be subsumed under the risk-management program. Ideally an organization ethics process would have an independent oversight relationship, such that it could serve as an early-warning mechanism for risk-management policies or proposals that have ethical implications.

A healthcare organization ethics program must directly influence risk management if it is to promote a dynamic ethical climate throughout the organization. Policies developed through risk management activities are increasingly strategic in nature. Strategic policies that will certainly change the structure of the HCO have the very real possibility of changing core attributes of the HCO if not considered carefully within the framework of the healthcare organization's ethical climate, which reflects those values endorsed by the HCO.

A healthcare organization ethics process can and must accommodate risk management. But it is through an organization ethics process, not a risk-management process, that organization goals and objectives can be integrated and balanced within the context of a comprehensive organization ethics program.

CONTINUOUS QUALITY-IMPROVEMENT PROGRAMS

Continuous quality-improvement programs have sought to ensure that patients receive consistently high quality and efficient care from the HCO. Quality is defined as something perceived by a customer and reached when the customer's needs and expectations concerning a product or a service are either met or surpassed. Customer expectations of a product or service are a function of a number of factors including the price, grade, and conformance to established standards of the product or service (Garrison & Noreen, 1997, p. 200).

The argument for incorporating quality standards into the daily functioning of the healthcare organization is a competitive argument that relies on some kind of measurement to determine whether objectives have been met. Organizations exist to provide goods or services, and the perception by the customer of the quality of that good or service will help determine the market share the organization in question enjoys. But quality depends on factors that can be identified and measured.

Ideas of how high quality can be achieved have been around since the 1911 publication of Frederick Taylor's *The Principles of Scientific Management*, in which he sought to reach this goal by inspection of the goods and services. This inspection approach was supplemented in the early 1980s when American business discovered the ideas of W. Edwards Deming and J.M. Juran. Deming and Juran, originators of the total quality management (TQM) movement, developed educational programs in quality management that, when implemented, resulted in staggering productivity gains for Japanese manufacturing. Deming's "14 Points to Quality" (Deming, 1981–1982), and Juran's insistence that 80 percent of quality defects are controllable by management (Juran & Gryna, 1980), became the basis of modern quality-improvement programs.

Continuous quality-improvement (CQI) is associated with the general management strategy of TQM. It shifts the focus of achieving quality to avoiding mistakes or preventing defects early on in the value-added activities of the organization. Underlying this idea is the notion that continuous small improvements in the way goods or services are produced, combined with the emphasis on avoiding mistakes or defects early in the activities which produce the product or service, will be cost-effective. These results will be reflected in customer satisfaction (Krajewski & Ritzman, 1993). Either a product or service of the same quality at a lower price or a quality-enhanced product or service at the same price will be perceived positively by consumers. This goal of maintaining the quality of healthcare services while holding down the rate of growth of costs is the primary objective of managed care.

The JCAHO made the shift away from the inspection model of quality assurance to CQI in 1992 when it introduced standards for CQI in its accreditation guidelines. This shift sparked a new round of debate about whether HCOs ought to focus their energies on improving the processes or improving the outcomes of healthcare delivery. The debate is to some extent spurious because of the interdependence of the two. Production methods or processes are in place precisely to produce predetermined outcomes, and the outcome desired will determine what processes are used. Nevertheless, both may carry ethical implications, so we seek below to differentiate between the process/production and consumption/outcomes approaches to achieving quality in the delivery of health care, although we recognize their interdependence.

The production/process approach to quality in the HCO

HCOs produce services for specific patient populations. They do this by using particular healthcare professionals, specific protocols, pathways, or processes, and specific types of equipment or technology housed in particular facilities. These are the raw materials that, when combined in predetermined processes, enable the HCO to fulfill its mission. Therefore, administrators for continuous quality-improvement programs will ask questions such as, What are our standards? Do our materials comply with these standards? Do the processes employed to accomplish desired outcomes do so in the most efficient way? What variation in standards is acceptable, what is not?

The question of variation in standards is an important one in considering how to achieve quality through the production process. Standards are in place to assure that the production process works as it was designed to work to produce desired outcomes. Variations from these standards are highlighted and addressed by those responsible, and these variances, because they can be identified, are measurable. But control through variation measurement has the potential to be rigid (and in most industries is necessarily rigid.) Control through variation measurement in health care may result in ethically problematic situations because flexibility may be bounded through inadequate variances or variances unsuited to a particular patient. We will discuss below two widely practiced healthcare management techniques, case management and utilization review, from the perspective of variance control.

A patient is assigned a case manager on admission to an HCO. The case manager helps coordinate the care the patient receives by interacting with the whole spectrum of the patient's caregivers and repeatedly checking assigned protocols against what has actually been done for the patient. If there is a variation between the two, the case manager immediately investigates and notifies those responsible for the variation. The case manager follows the patient's progress through an HCO from entry to exit with the goal of ensuring that the patient receives appropriate and allowable care. Hence costs and protocols associated with that patient's stay in the HCO can be monitored from entry to exit. The expectation is that by monitoring and evaluating each step of the patient's progress through the HCO, costs and quality outcomes can be better controlled and assured. Case management attempts to achieve both cost control and desirable and appropriate outcomes throughout the process of delivering health care by controlling the variance between a standard of optimum care, or "best care," and actual care. The difficulty is that "best care" is increasingly being defined for the whole patient population— not the individual.

Another process/production example of variance control is utilization review. The resources that were used in the care of a specific patient are measured and compared to a benchmark established earlier by the HCO as the average resources required for that particular illness or injury. The utilization review flags those occurrences of either underutilization or overutilization of resources associated with a particular outcome. Whether the case is investigated depends on the judgment of the utilization review manager. Although utilization review is retroactive, it provides measures for the manager of what was achieved at what cost, thus allowing the manager to make appropriate future interventions in the delivery of future health care.

The use of management techniques such as case management and utilization review means in practice that the flexibility, autonomy, and authority of the healthcare professional and the patient will be reduced. Healthcare professionals are guided through the treatment decisions they make for their patients by reference to standardized guidelines, which are based on information received from projects that seek to correlate treatment outcomes with treatment costs. An example is the National Committee for Quality Assurance's Health Plan Employer Data and Information Set (HEDIS 3.0) which provides plan-to-plan comparisons on a variety of different measures ranging from a plan's financial performance to quality of care to utilization of services.

Utilization review and case management could pose conflicting situations for the quality improvement manager. The manager is not only concerned with the process of achieving desired patient outcomes, but with the organizational goal of cost control. The individual patient who may require treatment more costly than the standard may pose a problem for the manager who is seeking a desirable outcome for the patient within the context of providing adequate patient care and keeping costs in line with predetermined objectives. Thus, the use of these CQI techniques may cause conflicts between the responsibilities and obligations of the HCO to particular patient-stakeholders, particularly when providing adequate care to a population of patients and economic stability are other important goals.

The outcomes/product approach to quality in the HCO

In a TQM/CQI model, the customer has been identified and the preferences and expectations of the customer understood by the organization. This allows the organization to try and meet and measure these preferences and expectations and so retain customer loyalty. TQM/CQI was designed to work in situations in which cost satisfaction and outcome satisfaction are tightly integrated in one customer or one kind of customer. If the payer for the product or service is also the user of the product or service, the customer, as both user and payer, can evaluate both and negotiate trade-offs by choosing between cost and outcome preferences, and so maximize and express a composite satisfaction index which can then be measured by the provider. In this model, the customer and provider share a common goal—highest quality for lowest cost—and results can be measured against expectations.

Society certainly expects the highest-quality health care for the lowest possible cost from the HCO. Measuring outcomes for healthcare delivery has not proved easy, however, and there is a vast literature debating various criteria for evaluation. For instance, there may be different results of a technology assessment comparing two medical procedures which takes only safety and efficacy of an intervention into consideration, and one which considers other criteria—cost related to benefit, patient discomfort, or inequitable distribution of the advantages of the two procedures (Fuchs & Garber, 1990). Cost-benefit analysis may yield differing results for the same procedures. Results may differ depending upon whether the criterion is the satisfaction of one patient or of entire populations of patients. The result is a remarkable paucity of objective data about the correlation between treatments and outcomes.

It has been argued that many patients are not technically competent to judge outcomes associated with healthcare interventions (Carson, Carson & Roe, 1995). The idea that a patient can die from a successful operation typically bewilders the nonmedical layperson. Therefore outcomes evaluations have tended to focus on the tangibles of healthcare delivery, such as facility attractiveness, reliability, waiting time, and so on. Applying these ideas to health care has resulted in numerous studies that have sought to understand consumer preferences and expectations. These studies are called outcomes or satisfaction studies.

The single most important dimension in TQM/CQI models is the identification of the customer. This identification allows the producer/provider to ascertain customer expectations. This question is not easily answered in the HCO. While there are manifold problems in designing outcomes studies in patient care, the fundamental problem, in our view, is the fact the customer in an HCO is not easily identified, or more precisely, there are two sets of customers the HCO is concerned with—the recipient of services (the consumer), and the payers of those services. Each set of customers has a different agenda, which leads to different preferences and expectations. Thus, each will define quality quite differently, and the criteria for meeting the differing expectations can be expected to diverge. The payer is interested in the dollar value of services received and so may encourage, if not require, the HCO with which it has a contractual relationship to monitor, report on, explain, or absorb the cost of variances. The patient, however, has a different view of the quality of healthcare services, though researchers are still unsure of how to evaluate that perception. It is important to note, though, that both sets of customers determine the HCO's overall viability and ability to survive. But because the expectations of the two groups are different, they may be incompatible in practice, or reconcilable only at the cost of compromise or dislocations.

Some of the dislocations in the current healthcare system can be understood by recalling our discussion of the contemporary HCO in Chapter 7. The relative power exerted within the HCO by the care providers and their patients, for whom medical efficacy and safety may be the primary determinants of quality, and the payers and administrators who prioritize cost considerations and results across populations, has internalized the conflict between two customer groups. The HCO must develop strategies to deal with possible conflicts between the two interests in order to fulfill its social mandate for high-quality care at the lowest possible cost.

Relationship of quality improvement to organization ethics

There are many techniques of modern management that have the potential for improving the morale and the ethical climate of the HCO, if they are used with a clear objective of furthering the effectiveness of the HCO for its primary purpose: providing excellent, or at least adequate health care to a patient population. Still, the fact that processes and outcomes are monitored and evaluated using TQM or CQI techniques does not necessarily mean that either processes or the outcomes associated with them meet the highest ethical standards. One may use TQM or CQI techniques to ensure unethical outcomes. Processes are monitored to ensure that defects or errors or variations from standards—those standards may be unethical—are picked up early. This enables those responsible to respond quickly to correct the error or defect and thus ensure that a desired and cost-effective outcome is achieved. In health care this is achieved through variance-control techniques such as case management and utilization review. But management tools do not necessarily ensure ethical processes or outcomes. They are merely that— management tools. Potential for conflicts of commitment in the processes of delivering health care arises, because the question of whether the patient or the payer is the ultimate customer of the HCO cannot be answered satisfactorily in every case. Processes are designed, modified, or eliminated depending on the outcomes desired by those who consume the product—and generally the consumer (customer) is the payer. If the HCO's ultimate customer is the payer, then the HCO will inevitably endorse healthcare processes that reflect the payer's expectations and these expectations may be skewed toward cost control. If the HCO's ultimate customer is the patient, then the HCO will endorse preferences that reflect patient expectations typically quality issues such as access to "best" care. We anticipate that the HCO will continue, at least in the near-term future, to continue to try to satisfy the expectations of these two sets of customers. But in a competitive market, the possibility for conflicting expectations will inevitably intensify. This is a strong argument for the implementation of a healthcare organization ethics program.

   Any outcome experienced by any patient who has been involved in a process of health care will reflect and influence the HCO's ethical climate (either positively or negatively). Through these processes, the patient (or surrogate or family) will interact with both healthcare and administrative professionals who each have roles and responsibilities they are obligated to fulfill. The healthcare organization ethics program and the goals it represents may help the organization balance its commitment to both sets of customers by referencing its healthcare processes within the organization's stated values. Additionally, it allows conflicts between both differing sets of customers, and individual patients, and standards of care to be made public and discussed with the aim of resolution in a forum that represents the interests and obligations of all stakeholders within the HCO.

Since programs that use the ideas of TQM and CQI cannot guarantee acceptable ethical processes and outcomes, a healthcare organization ethics program should not be subsumed to the goals of quality-improvement programs. Conversely, a healthcare organization ethics program may work to inform quality-improvement managers of potential areas of conflict between the goals of the organization that will be determined by the two sets of customers the organization serves, and the values endorsed by the HCO.

CONCLUSION

Corporate compliance, risk management, and quality improvement are important to the HCOs in very specific and focused ways, and, as a result, most HCOs currently have programs designed to achieve the goals discussed above. An organization ethics program has its own set of goals. Since, by definition, its goals affect all activities within the HCO, these goals should not be subsumed under other program goals. It is therefore imperative to distinguish between other programs and the goals of a healthcare organization ethics program. If we clearly distinguish the various programs, the HCO will be able to situate these programs within the context of the values endorsed by the organization. In this way the diverse and important goals of these program activities will be initiated and supported within the larger context of reinforcing and enhancing the ethical climate of the organization.

Our objective in this chapter has been to discuss these program goals and differentiate them from the goal of the healthcare organization ethics program. Its goal is not primarily to protect the organization from the fines associated with wrongdoing or to promote a compliance climate within the organization. Nor is its key aim to ensure that the organization is protected or gains through the assumption or avoidance of certain types of risk, nor is it variance control of the processes and outcomes of health care. The implementation of the health care organization ethics program should provide a set of processes that protects the integrity of the organization as the organization seeks to fulfill these legitimate but differing objectives. The program should provide a forum for discussion and resolution when legal, strategic, or quality issues clash with each other or with the stated and unstated values that comprise the organization's mission and are reflected in its activities.

11

Organization Ethics Activities
and Their Evaluation

Any activity undertaken by an organization should be consistent with the mission and goals of that organization. If it is important to an organization that it have a positive ethical climate, the effective functioning of the organization's ethical processes will not only influence but also, at times, *direct* activities critical to the fulfillment of the organization's mission.

An organization ethics program engages in various activities, including policy review and development, communication activities, education, and in some instances, consultation. To strengthen an organization's ethical climate, the activities that are designed to affect it must be evaluated to determine whether the organization ethics program is fulfilling its purposes.

The structure of the organization ethics program and the activities it supports are not complex, and appropriate evaluations do not require complex evaluation designs or strategies. But inappropriate approaches may provide useless or even misleading information. For this reason we begin this chapter with a brief discussion of the purposes of evaluation and an overview of the commonly accepted evaluation approaches used in health care. Those responsible for the organization ethics program will want to know whether it can fulfill the goals it has set itself. We therefore follow the general discussion of evaluation methods with a recapitulation of the organization ethics program itself in conjunction with possible approaches to evaluating it and its goals in the second segment of this chapter. In the third section we discuss in some detail several of the activities that may be critical to the success of the organization ethics program: policy review and development, communication activities, and education. We offer suggestions as to how each can be evaluated.

It is clear that the organization ethics process needs some way of being alerted to possible issues that arise in the ongoing function of the organization and some means of communication between stakeholder groups. There is some controversy over whether this should take the form of a "consultation service" similar to the consultation service offered by many patient care ethics committees. Even if the organization ethics program offers a consultation service, it must be able to deal with ethically problematic *systems or processes* as well as with individual conflicts. This will involve a different approach to problem resolution than that currently taken by many committees which offer clinical ethics consultation. In the fourth section of this chapter we suggest an approach to problem identification and resolution that could be instituted by the organization ethics program. The chapter concludes with a discussion of how the organization ethics program and the activities it supports relate to certain widely accepted management and professional practices.

PURPOSE OF EVALUATION

We evaluate programs and processes for several reasons: to determine the baseline conditions before instituting a change, to measure the consequences of change, to justify retaining or altering programs, or to gather information for organizational purposes. Before embarking on the actual design of an evaluation it is necessary to know exactly what activity is being evaluated and why. The evaluator needs to begin his or her task with clear answers to these questions as well as a clear understanding of what questions the evaluation is expected to answer. These questions are often divided into the categories of access, efficiency, and quality (Fox, 1996, p. 117).

Access has to do with the target population of the activity in question. No matter how worthwhile an activity, if the target population is not reached then that activity fails to accomplish its objective (p. 118). The most effective clinical ethics processes, for instance, are available to a wide range of clinicians, patients, and family members. Efficiency questions concern the cost/benefit ratio of the activity in question. No matter how worthwhile it is, an activity will not be supported if it is prohibitively expensive (p. 118). In what follows, we will subsume questions of access and efficiency under the category of quality, which asks how well the activity under examination accomplishes its objective.

Three widely accepted approaches to evaluation of quality consider *outcomes*, *process*, and *structure* (p. 118). *Outcomes* are the consequences or results—the product—of a process or program. To evaluate outcomes, the actual results can be compared to desired outcomes or previous outcomes and the difference measured in some way. *Satisfaction* evaluations are a common and well-known version of outcome studies based on one type of outcome—the satisfaction of the affected stakeholder after experiencing the activity under question. Satisfaction studies seek to correlate the outcome of an activity to some measure of perceived quality. The gap between perceived quality and desired quality can be measured quantitatively or descriptively, depending on the context of the evaluation.

Process evaluation is applied to an activity or series of activities by which a desired result is accomplished. Process evaluations—often referred to as *efficiency studies* or *process analyses*—measure the effectiveness of processes by investigating the way they work. A process evaluation may compare a specific activity or series of activities to standards that have been agreed upon for the process in question, or it may be used to reengineer or redesign the activity under consideration (Garrison & Noreen, 1997, p. 18). The central question asked in a process evaluation is whether the process under consideration can be improved.

Structure refers to the resources employed to support a process and its organization. An evaluation of the structure of a process will look at issues such as personnel and equipment employed, training, time involved, facilities needed, and so forth. A structure evaluation will try to identify all the resources used to support a process and try to answer the question of whether these resources are sufficient to achieve the goals of the process. Structure evaluations are often the starting point for efficiency or process evaluations (Garrison & Noreen, 1997, p. 184).

It is notoriously difficult to agree upon and define appropriate outcomes measurement in health care (Eddy, 1998). A number of factors contribute to this difficulty but it is especially true when one is trying to measure an outcome for which a whole range of possibilities is permissible (Thier & Gelijns, 1998). For instance, clinical ethics consultations have been extremely difficult to evaluate, since even a very efficient process may occur in situations where the satisfaction of the participants may be more determined by the difficulties of the case in question than by the intervention of the consultants (Fox & Arnold, 1996). But because process, structure, and outcomes are so intimately linked—a desired outcome will be influenced by process and structure and vice versa—in many instances, a process or a structure approach to evaluation can serve as a proxy for an outcomes evaluation (Eddy, 1998, p. 17).

In the following discussion we suggest whichever evaluation approach seems most likely to yield useful information.

EVALUATING AN ORGANIZATION ETHICS PROGRAM

The organization ethics program is charged with the responsibility of enhancing and supporting a consistent positive ethical climate within the organization. The resources it has at its disposal will determine what activities the committee can support. Thus, a structure approach can be helpful in evaluating the program as a whole.

The structural standards may have been agreed upon within the organization, or may have been developed outside the organization. For instance, an organization ethics program may seek to evaluate its composition, its location within the organization, and the types of activities it supports, against the standards recommended by the Virginia Bioethics Network (see Appendix 1). In Chapter 9 we explored characteristics of the organization ethics program that we believe are important to ensure its success in meeting its goals. There we recommend making the organization ethics program the responsibility of a committee rather than an individual, discuss its location near the top of the organization's hierarchy, delimit areas of decision-making authority, and include responsibility for reporting functions. We made suggestions concerning the composition of the committee, some channels of communication, and some recommended activities. The model developed in Chapter 9 can be also used as the basis for a structure evaluation. Questions that persons responsible for the program may ask include:

1. What formal structures have been developed to initiate and advance the organization ethics program?
2. To whom does the organization ethics program report? Why was that person or group chosen?
3. Who is involved with the program? Do these persons represent the major stakeholders, departments, and activities of the HCO? Who leads the program?
4. What issues does the organization ethics committee address? Ethics? Compliance? Accreditation? Profiling? Contractual relationships?
5. Is the organization ethics committee advisory only? If not, what decision-making authority does the committee have? In what areas does the committee have this authority? Why should the committee have this authority?
6. What general activities does the process support? Mission? Codes of ethics? Policy review? Policy development? Communication activities? Education? Does the committee have a consultation service that can respond to stakeholder concerns? Should it do so? What alternative response mechanism does it employ?
7. How is the program itself structured? Into various subcommittees? Do these subcommittees include a patient care subcommittee? A management ethics subcommittee? A professional ethics subcommittee? A corporate compliance subcommittee? Should the program have community representation?
8. Are reporting functions adequate to ensure appropriate and complete communication between the subcommittees? Does the program have an adequate administrative infrastructure?

9. Does the program have a budget? Who supplies it, and what does it include? Does it include released time for the members?
10. Have persons assigned to the program been allocated sufficient time to accomplish the activities for which they are responsible?

By evaluating the program against previously developed internal or external standards the HCO can gain an appreciation of what it may or may not be able to accomplish and how easy or difficult it may be to accomplish its goals. For this reason, we recommend that the program evaluate its structure and the resources it has at its disposal before attempting any major changes.

GOAL OF THE ORGANIZATION ETHICS PROGRAM

If the primary objectives of an organization ethics committee are to support and enhance an overall positive ethical climate, achievement of that goal should be evaluated. In this instance the best evaluation approach is an outcomes evaluation consisting of measuring an actual outcome against a desired outcome.

It is necessary to be very precise about what is meant by "supporting and enhancing a positive ethical climate" before an outcomes evaluation can be designed. As we have discussed above, the ethical climate is measured by the extent to which the stakeholders in an organization understand the ethical values, norms, and expectations of the organization, and how well they perceive the organization lives up to those standards. The values, norms, and expectations of the organization's stakeholders (the real ethical climate) can be measured against the organization's stated values, norms, and expectations (the stated ethical climate) and the differences analyzed. One appropriate outcomes evaluation could be an organization-wide survey of stakeholders in the organization. Such a survey could help measure the effectiveness of the organization ethics program in closing the gap between the stated ethical standards of the organization and its effectiveness in meeting them.

A survey of this sort will consist of questions designed to explore some of the following general issues:

1. How general is the awareness in the organization of the contents of the HCO's mission statement and code of ethics?
2. What are the values that the organization supports?
3. How important are the mission and the code of ethics to the organization?
4. How effective is the code of ethics? Does it guide both individual and organization decision making?

Frank Navran, a consultant for the AHA's organization ethics initiative, described in Chapter 1, calls this an "ethics inventory." It can be offered both before and after policies, procedures, or education aimed at enhancing the ethical climate have been implemented and communicated. There are strong arguments that an ethics inventory should be taken before the organization embarks on any sort of activity that has as its goal some effect on the ethical climate of the organization. It may very well highlight areas of confusion or areas of potential conflict among different individuals, different levels of individuals, and different groups of stakeholders. For example, it may be helpful to survey different levels of clinicians and compare the results with a similar survey of different levels of managers. Such a survey could indicate how widely these two groups diverge in their values, norms, and expectations as measured both against the stated organization values and each other. It may also indicate a consensus or divergence between the two groups at different levels in the organization hierarchy. An ethics inventory should, at a minimum, provide the organization ethics program with an indication of the degree of divergence between the organization's stated ethical objectives and the actual perception of its ethical climate. This can help focus the activities of the organization ethics program.

ACTIVITIES OF THE ORGANIZATION ETHICS PROGRAM

An organization ethics program will support certain activities to achieve its goal. These activities include policy review and development, communication activities, and education. The organization ethics program may also support consultation activities.

It is not usually necessary to evaluate all the activities that the program initiates. Any program must assign priorities to the work it undertakes, given the time and resource constraints under which the committee operates. If one activity has the potential to have a much greater impact on the ethical climate than another, that activity justifies a much more painstaking evaluation. It may be necessary to substitute one type of evaluation for another or to use more than one approach in evaluating the activity under consideration. Therefore, the following discussion of possible evaluation approaches for these activities should be considered a general guide rather than a recommendation that each and every activity be evaluated with the same degree of detail and attention.

Policy development and review

One of the first tasks assigned to the organization ethics program will likely be to review the organization's mission statement, values statement, and organization code of ethics. This task can be a way of evaluating the congruence of these statements with the actual or desired ethical climate of the organization. It is also the first step towards meeting the JCAHO's organization ethics standards.

Contractual relationships direct interactions between the organization and those outside the organization. These interactions and the effects they have are a clear measure of what the organization will do to fulfill its mission within the values it espouses. If the HCO is serious about acting according to its espoused ethical standards, the organization ethics program can play an important role in scrutinizing the HCO's relationships with managed care organizations and provider groups that interact directly with patients. We anticipate that in addition to reviewing internal policies, the organization ethics process will sooner or later need tools to review contractual relationships with other organizations and stakeholders outside the organization. This review would consider whether the conditions of those relationships were consistent with the organization's mission and code of ethics. Whether the organization ethics program also assumes the role of reviewing departmental or functional policies will vary, depending on what role the organization ethics process plays in each individual organization.

Policy development and policy review are coordinate processes. In the process of reviewing existing policies it is possible to find that they are insufficient to meet current needs of the organization. Policy development can also be prompted in response to a new or critical situation, or because a certain activity has become important enough to require a new policy or a change to an existing policy. Since policy review and policy development are so similar, we can use similar approaches to evaluating them. We begin first with questions that can form the basis of a structure evaluation of a policy review/policy development activity:

1. Who is leading the policy review/development effort? What support does the designated leader have?
2. What areas of the organization are affected? Should these affected areas be represented on the review/development team?
3. What reporting functions should be required?
4. When should these reporting functions be invoked?
5. What budget is necessary?
6. What expertise will be needed?

An outcomes evaluation of a policy review and development effort might seek to measure whether the objectives were met. This involves formulating questions on the specific goal of the effort and measuring the change induced by the policy change:

1. What were the specific objectives of the policy review/development effort?
2. How is success defined?
3. How can success be best measured? By monitoring? Audits? Surveys?

Communication

Internal and external communications are crucial to the morale, reputation, and ethical consistency of an organization. People and other organizations cannot align their values, norms, and expectations to those of an HCO unless they *know* what those values, norms, and expectations are and how they are expressed in various situations that the organization and its stakeholders confront. If an organization ethics program is to be successful, it must take communication activities very seriously. Communication activities are distinguished from educational activities because communication is an ongoing process rather than a series of discrete events designed to achieve specific educational or informational objectives. For example, an educational program may seek to acquaint some of its internal stakeholders with tests for ethical decision making. A communication activity, on the other hand, may give all stakeholders (external and internal) examples of how these tests are used in practice and what they mean to the ethical climate.

All organizations have vehicles for communication with internal and external stakeholders. While informal communication among stakeholders is important, it is unstructured and cannot be assessed within a formal structure, and so will not be discussed here. Formal communication vehicles include organization newsletters, public relations and media facilities and events, marketing departments, and, increasingly, e-mail facilities.

Each can be of use to the organization ethics program as it seeks to communicate to *all* stakeholders the values of the organization.

A structure evaluation will consider the resources needed to communicate. This will involve answering such questions as:

1. Who will be responsible for the communication activities?
2. What support will that person have?

A process evaluation of communication vehicles will consider:

1. Which stakeholder group does each communication vehicle target?
2. Which vehicle is most effective in communicating the "message"? Is there a vehicle that is perceived as more credible than another? Is there a point at which these vehicles break down in communicating?
3. Is communication effective in reaching all primary stakeholders?

An outcomes evaluation will consider:

1. Has the message reached the target audience?
2. Has it affected the perceptions or behavior of the target audience in the way in which it was intended?

Education

Since every stakeholder of an organization makes decisions throughout her association with the organization, any attempt by the organization to alter the organization's values, ethical standards, or implementation processes needs the participation of *all* of the organization's stakeholders. Stakeholders, at a minimum, need education about the stated ethical standards of the organization, its sanctions for specific behavior, and simple models for ethical decision making. The organization ethics process might offer different levels of education to its stakeholders depending upon their decision making roles.

Most HCOs have some sort of program for new employee orientation. This orientation should incorporate material about the ethical standards of the organization and the policies and procedures that support it. An easy-to-use model for ethical decision making could be introduced to new employees at this time. This model should be simple, easy to learn, easy to teach, and quite effective. For instance, one common and effective test that an employee could apply to an ethically troublesome decision is whether the chosen alternative is one that the employee and the HCO could live with if it were publicly exposed. See Appendices 2 and 3 for two such models.

An effective process should involve increasing numbers of stakeholders in its projects. As the decision-making authority of various stakeholder groups increases it may be appropriate to acquaint those stakeholders with a more complex picture of the impact of decisions on the organization's ethical climate. For instance, in Chapter 10 we discussed the increasing importance of risk management within the HCO and the potential effect risk-management decisions may have on the ethical climate of the organization. As risk management makes more and more complex decisions aimed at helping the organization gain through appropriate strategies, the ethical implications of those decisions need to be considered. It may well be that the organization ethics program will need to support ongoing education to enhance awareness of emerging issues and their ethical impact.

Continuing medical and nursing education programs in many HCOs already provide educational activities that can be expanded to include different constituencies within the organization. Many such programs already have evaluations in place that can be used by the organization ethics program.

A structure evaluation of educational activities will consider:

1. Who identifies, initiates, and oversees educational content for the various stakeholders? What qualifications should that individual have to bring a strong sense of authority/credibility to the project?
2. Who teaches desired educational content? What qualifications for educators are necessary?

3. Should education be required? Is it appropriate that all stakeholders be exposed to the specific education content envisioned?
4. When should particular educational content be presented?
5. How should the desired education be delivered? New employee orientation? Seminars? Newsletters? Videos?

An outcomes evaluation determines whether educational objectives were achieved. This involves considering whether stakeholder perceptions have been altered or stakeholder knowledge increased by the educational activity. This involves asking:

1. What are the educational objectives?
2. What defines achievement of education objectives?
3. What is the best way of measuring achievement? Participant knowledge before and after responses? Surveys? Monitoring a specific situation? Audits?

RESPONDING TO STAKEHOLDER CONCERNS: IDENTIFICATION AND RESPONSE

All of the possible activities of an organization ethics process—policy review and development, communication, and education—are designed and implemented in response to a perceived need or problem. Evaluation of these activities assumes that the problem or need has been identified, alternatives considered, and decisions made concerning the most appropriate way to address the identified problem. Identifying problems and providing ways of addressing them is analogous to the activities of a consultant, whose role is to identify problems and suggest ways to solve them. Thus, the organization ethics program has an implicit consulting role whether or not the program explicitly includes consultation among its functions. However controversial, it is a role that should be considered carefully by the program.

The task of identifying ethical obstacles to excellent organizational function and responding to them is the major task of the organization ethics program. We offer below a hypothetical situation in which an ethically problematic outcome is brought to the attention of the organization ethics program and suggest a *process* evaluation of the committee's response. We discuss the important steps an organization ethics program can take in order to resolve it. Our example may not apply in every respect, depending on the role the organization ethics program assumes and the resources it has at its disposal. We hope, however, that it will acquaint readers unfamiliar with problem-solving devices and systems analysis tools with their possible application in this context.

1. The program identifies what seems to be an ethically inappropriate activity or outcome.

An ethically problematic activity or outcome can be brought to the attention of the organization ethics program any number of ways: through policy review, review of contracts, through requests for assistance from the patient care ethics subcommittee, by one of the members of the committee itself, or by any other stakeholder in the organization. The identification of a possible problem is itself no easy task. It presupposes that there are well-advertised routes of access to the committee available to a wide range of constituencies within the organization. It presupposes as well that there has been a process of ethical education sensitizing the various stakeholders to what ethical conduct the organization expects. The ability to foresee problematic ethical consequences from current decisions is one which will need to be cultivated within the HCO.

2. A designated individual or committee decides whether the identified activity or outcome falls within the parameters tolerated by the organization by consulting the mission statement and its supporting policies.

This decision can only be made if the designated agent has complete and thorough knowledge of the organization's values, norms, and expectations. This is a strong argument for the committee organization ethics program to be located at the highest level in the organization, since it is here that those expectations are determined. It also suggests persons appointed to this problem-solving group should receive appropriate education before addressing issues which may be of central importance.

3. If the problematic activity or outcome is not within the parameters tolerated by the organization the committee should consider the scope of the problem.

Is the source of the problem easily addressed? If the specific issues at stake are not easily identifiable the committee must consider whether it has the resources and skills to properly identify the specific problem, or will need to go outside the committee, or possibly outside the organization, for help. Whatever the results of that decision, the committee must consider resource issues. These issues will include financial costs, timeliness, confidentiality, conflict-of-interest issues, and oversight.

4. Once the source of the problem has been satisfactorily identified, the committee will need to identify and evaluate alternatives to correct the problem.

Identifying alternatives may be accomplished through the use of "what if" analysis. The committee needs to walk through each activity or decision to identify other changes that may occur and their potential effect on the desired outcome. Any change must be evaluated for its implications for the mission of the organization, its ethical standards, and the costs and legal ramifications of the change.

Consideration of alternatives by the committee is generally beneficial. The organization ethics program addresses structural or organization-wide issues, and it is very likely that a system-wide problem will affect more than one department or function, as will any proposed change. It is at this point that the committee has the opportunity to build a consensus for recommending or implementing a change. This consensus will contribute to making any changes in the least disruptive fashion. Notice that consensus does not require complete agreement on every point nor on every issue. Rather the goal is to find areas of agreement that the committee can use in building further consensus.

5. Choose among possible alternatives.

The criteria by which the committee decides to either recommend or implement an alternative do not change. The committee's responsibility is to maintain and enhance a positive ethical climate within the organization, and that responsibility governs the choice of an alternative.

6. Implement any chosen changes

Implementation of any change will almost certainly be the responsibility of the department in which the source of the problem was found. However, it should occur with the cooperation and full knowledge of other departments or functions which may be affected by the change.

7. The change should be monitored to ensure its success.

Monitoring may be considered to be the responsibility of those who are affected by the change. However, the organization ethics program should be involved in some way—probably through those persons who are responsible for recommending the change. Unforeseen consequences or changes in circumstance may require that the problem be revisited.

Each step presented above represents an activity or series of activities. Because changes in one or more systems have the potential to affect the mission and ethical climate of the organization, the organization ethics program may develop mechanisms formally or informally to evaluate each of the steps and the overall process.

RELATIONSHIP OF ORGANIZATION ETHICS
TO OTHER MANAGEMENT PRACTICES

There are some obvious parallels between an organization ethics program as we have described it and other widely accepted management tools, such as total quality management (see Chapter 10). Both TQM and the organization ethics program seek to affect the climate of the organization by building on the values it endorses. Both recognize that while success is not ensured by the involvement of top management, such involvement is a necessary precondition of any success. Both recognize that departmental boundaries and levels can be impediments to success and that it may be necessary to cross these boundaries in order to achieve their respective goals. Both recognize that some sort of measurement or evaluation is crucial in order to determine the success or failure of a proposed change or activity. Both recognize the importance of communication, and both recognize that conflict resolution among stakeholders must be built on some kind of consensus.

In some ways, the organization ethics program can be thought of as a "quality circle" which is one technique used by those seeking to implement concepts of TQM within their organization. These groups were widely used during the 1970s and 1980s as a means of improving the quality of output. Management and "front-line" workers (workers who guide or direct or who are involved in the production process) met on a regularly scheduled basis to brainstorm ways to improve the production processes. One result of these meetings was that each group better understood the objectives and needs of the other, thus allowing some consensus between these disparate groups on what was desirable and what was achievable. This is one goal of the organization ethics program.

The formation of the organization ethics program parallels that of a quality circle, in that its members may have disparate objectives or a different set of priorities within the context of a common goal. Those responsible for the activities of an organization ethics program, like those in a quality circle, will often include both management and front-line employees, who in the HCO are professional clinicians, and should include patient representatives as well.

An organization ethics program has the potential to bring to the HCO other benefits that may not be directly related to its central goal. The committee or group responsible for the organization ethics program will ideally include representatives from all critical areas in the HCO. The committee structure offers its members an avenue of communication, a means of ensuring that members from all critical areas understand the objectives and processes by which the organization fulfills its mission. It offers the possibility of a continuous review of the constraints within which each representative operates, with the possibility of addressing some of those constraints. It offers the possibility of consensus building at the highest levels that in turn lead to increased management, professional, and nonprofessional employee confidence in the leadership of the organization. Thus, the discussions and considerations of the organization ethics committee may improve understanding and decision making in other areas that can positively affect the performance of the HCO.

It is estimated that climate changes in organizations can take as much as ten years (Wilhelm, 1992, p. 72). Effecting positive changes in organizations requires patience, constant reinforcement, and resources. Appropriate use of evaluation tools can help focus the organization ethics program, and highlight areas of potential conflict. They can be used as indicators of efficiency and a guide to self-correction for the program. Good evaluation methods can significantly reduce the amount of time needed to positively affect the organization's ethical climate and can be a source of reassurance not only for the persons most directly involved in the program but for all managers, professionals, other employees, and external stakeholders.

CONCLUSION

What do we want an organization ethics program in an HCO to accomplish, and what will it need to do it? How can we show its effectiveness to the various parties in the organization responsible for providing the resources it needs to function? We want a forum for the discussion of actual and potential ethical conflicts that might arise from, or accompany, the many decisions an HCO must make in dealing with the contemporary changing conditions of healthcare delivery. We want a way to prioritize the multiple and occasionally conflicting values which the HCO seeks to realize, and mechanisms which give some hope of integrating HCO activities around those values. We want a unified voice, a united front, which can speak for, as well as to, the various internal and external stakeholders of the HCO. Not every institution will adopt the same model of an organization ethics process, nor will every institution want to entrust it with the full range of functions we have suggested. But whatever its goals and functions, some means of evaluation to justify its role in the institution must be an integral part of its implementation. We have offered in this chapter various strategies of evaluation appropriate for both the initial stages of an organization ethics program and its ongoing operation. The ultimate goal of an organization ethics program is to forge a powerful voice that can help the stakeholders, all of whom wish to have their interests acknowledged and their needs met, to work in tandem instead of against each other.

12

Conclusion

We have defined organization ethics, we have applied various ethics approaches to organization ethics, and we have called attention to numerous divergent forces that have a negative impact on healthcare organizations today. Before moving to the practical task of instituting organization ethics programs, let us summarize our argument.

In Chapter 1 we suggested some provisional definitions of organization ethics. There we quoted the Virginia Bioethics Network definition:

> Organization ethics consists of a process to address ethical issues associated with patient care, with the business, financial, and management areas of healthcare organizations, as well as with professional, educational, and contractual relationships affecting the operation of the HCO.

It is difficult, however, to spell out the ethics of an *organization*, in contrast to the ethics of the individuals, such as professionals, managers, clinicians, and patients, who act independently and as agents for an organization. To begin, we argued in Chapter 2 that organizations, like individuals, are moral agents, but unlike individual people they are collective moral agents that depend on other agents (individuals and groups of individuals) to act on their behalf. We discussed the shortcomings of thinking about organizations as self-contained, closed, formal entities, analogous to autonomous individuals. Such a consideration fails to account for individual input into the organization. It conflates goal achievements with positive moral outcomes, and there are few avenues for external evaluation either of the roles and role responsibilities of those acting on behalf of the organization, or of the organization's own mission, activities, goals, and achievements. To avoid these difficulties, one must appeal to principles or moral minimums that are not merely self-referential.

A more fruitful approach to thinking about organizations, at least HCOs, is to define them as open systems. In HCOs, as in other open systems, there is no single reference point or phenomenon that characterizes all elements of a HCO. While activities of a particular HCO may be located in a particular healthcare center or set of centers, HCO stakeholders are an ever changing group of individuals who have roles and role responsibilities both within and outside the organization. Healthcare professionals, for example, even if they are full-time employees of a particular HCO, have professional commitments to the associations through which they are accredited, as well as various other roles outside the organization. Moreover, as we have demonstrated in Chapters 6 and 7, the HCO interacts with a variety of ever-shifting external stakeholders such as payers, lawyers, accountants, suppliers, government regulators, and the community. HCOs exist in a legal, economic, and political environment and under media scrutiny that creates an external climate that affects the operation and even character of the HCO. Therefore, one should think of a HCO as a dynamic set of structures, processes, and activities that continuously interacts with its internal and external stakeholders within a community and in a changing political, economic, and social regulatory system and climate.

As open systems, organizations, like individuals, have goal-defined roles and role obligations. All of these make up organizational role morality. In the case of healthcare organizations, their constitutive goal is to provide health care. Their societally expected primary role obligations are to do just that, and to do it well, for a particular population. We evaluate HCOs in terms of how well the organization embeds processes that emulate professional excellence, whom it serves and how well it provides healthcare services to the population in question. As in evaluating individuals in their roles, we evaluate an organization and organization climate not merely on how consistently, coherently, and adequately they achieve their self-defined goals, but by criteria external to the organization: excellence in healthcare service and delivery, and positive health-related outcomes.

It is tempting to approach organization ethics by appealing to other areas of applied ethics, e.g., clinical ethics, business ethics, or professional ethics. Indeed, as we argued in Chapter 3, clinical ethics, with its focus on patient care, helps us to think about the centrality of patient care for any healthcare organization. However, while this focus is critical in thinking about the ethics of healthcare organizations, it is insufficient as an approach to organization ethics. Clinical ethics tends to be preoccupied with the clinician and her relationships to the patient, in the first instance, an individual patient. But HCOs are complex organizations with a managerial structure, a number of stakeholders, and they serve a patient population. A preoccupation with a single patient is usually inadequate to explain and evaluate how an HCO serves its population. A clinical ethics approach, by itself, often pays insufficient attention to other stakeholders, in particular nonprofessional managers, and more significantly, payers.

What we demonstrated in Chapter 3, however, is that by using clinical ethics as an analogue, one can begin to think about clinical issues from an organizational perspective. This is not merely because clinical ethics issues have organizational implications. It is because other elements of clinical ethics contribute to developing an organization ethics perspective. As we pointed out, clinical ethics is not so much a distinct theory but has developed as a practical response to the mandates of medical ethics, bioethics, and public policy. Clinical ethics is best described as a set of strategies or procedures for adjudicating between differing perceptions of a given clinical situation, very much a "process" rather than a "normative" definition. Similarly, one way to think about organization ethics is that it is a process or set of strategies for adjudicating differing stakeholder points of view in an organization (see VBN definition). In a clinical setting this adjudication is usually carried out by an institutional ethics committee within an HCO, through educational endeavors, or by healthcare ethics consultants. In parallel, the work of an HCO organization ethics committee could and should take such an approach, now expanded to include issues in organizational, business, and professional ethics. Even so, as we concluded in Chapter 3, one needs a more comprehensive perspective, process, or theory concerning organization ethics to fill out the analogue.

Because of its interest in organizations, in particular corporations, business ethics appears to be the natural source of a robust theory of organization ethics. As we argued in Chapter 4, however, one must take care not to conflate HCOs with other kinds of corporations, nor to imagine that healthcare "commodities" are identical to other market-exchanged commodities. The vulnerability of most healthcare patients, the separation of payer from patient, the crucial necessity of professional excellence, and the lurking commitment to community access complicate the healthcare organization. Asymmetries of information, supply and demand, and pricing further complicate attempts to commodify health care in any straightforward manner. A standard stakeholder model does not capture the priority of patients and patient populations as primary stakeholders, the importance of professional excellence, or the ever present commitment to the patient population.

Still, as we suggested, a reworked stakeholder model is helpful in thinking through organizational issues in health care. The normative core of stakeholder theory allows us to analyze individual stakeholders (professionals, managers, patients) *and* organizations (HCOs, payers, government) as moral agents, both internally in their role accountability relationships and externally by more general moral criteria. One begins with the organization: the HCO and its mission.

One then prioritizes its stakeholders and its value-creating activities in terms of this mission, placing patients and patient population health first, followed by professional excellence (without which an HCO cannot serve its mission nor succeed), then organizational viability, community access, and public health. Thus stakeholder theory enables us to lay out the moral parameters for internal and external evaluation of various stakeholders, both individual and organizational, their roles and obligations, and set the guidelines for adjudicating organizational issues. But by itself, it too, is inadequate for a full-blown approach to organization ethics.

Healthcare professionals account for the core of organizational excellence. Without good professionals dedicated to their work, a healthcare organization will not succeed. Indeed, one can make a strong case that healthcare professionals are one of the two sets of crucial stakeholders in HCOs. The Hippocratic oath states that the protection of the patient is the first priority, and the codes of every healthcare profession stipulate that patient welfare and well-being are the primary objectives of any healthcare professional. Even the American College of Healthcare Executives specifies in its code that one of the key objectives of healthcare managers is to "enhance the overall quality of life, dignity, and well-being of every individual needing healthcare services."

Still, neither the codes of healthcare professionals or of healthcare managers focuses on the organization as a moral agent. Their codes do not adequately take into account the myriad of organizational stakeholders nor the reciprocal obligations between an HCO and those to whom it is accountable. Professional ethics provides the necessary ingredients for the content of an HCO mission statement, and reinforces the mandate for professional excellence, critical for healthcare delivery. But as these codes are presently articulated, they are not sufficient, by themselves, for a full fledged notion of organization ethics.

Given the organizational dimensions and analogies of clinical ethics, business ethics, and professional ethics, what roles do they play in the ethics of an organization—in particular, a healthcare organization? Let us assume that healthcare organizations are open systems that interact with various stakeholders within an external political, social, and even religious climate that affects their structure, culture, internal climate, and scope of activities. However that external climate is construed, what is characteristic about healthcare organizations is that by definition, their primary mission is, or should be, providing excellent, or at least adequate, health care to the patient populations they serve. A second part of the mission is, or should be, to encourage, promote, and preserve professional excellence among all those working with or for the HCO. Interestingly, clinical ethics as we have described it, an expanded stakeholder model, professional ethics, and managerial ethics as expressed by the ACHE, all agree on these two points. Each of these approaches to health care also envisions a commitment to community and public health as part of the mission of any HCO, although differently prioritized in particular circumstances. There is another important area in which there is some overlapping consensus. While HCOs may be for-profit, not-for-profit, community-run, or charitable institutions, in the present climate of limited resources, every HCO in the United States has to be economically viable, that is, each has to survive in a competitive economic climate. Even those HCOs that depend on community, religious, or charitable contributions find themselves under pressure to be more efficient, to be budget conscious, and to think carefully about to whom and how they provide health care. Healthcare professionals, clinicians, and patients as well as managers find themselves increasingly economically accountable. Thus *a* priority of any HCO, and one about which there should be some consensus among healthcare professionals, managers, payers, and patients, is to be economically viable. Professionals and patients will place this as *third or fourth* among the priorities of a HCO; managers might disagree, but the point is that there is consensus that economic viability cannot be dismissed or ignored. Figure 12.1 illustrates this consensus.

If the key stakeholders in HCOs are patients (individual or populations), professionals, managers, and payers, and if there is some overlapping consensus on basic healthcare priorities between clinical ethics, stakeholder theory, healthcare professional codes, and the code of the ACHE, a comprehensive organizational perspective should be able to integrate and protect these perspectives. From this consensus we conclude that as moral agent HCOs have certain socially, clinically, economically, and professionally defined roles:

1. The health and well-being of patients and patient populations
2. Professional excellence
3. Long-term organizational viability including economic stability
4. Community access
5. Public health.

Given these roles, we can now judge the value-creating activities and organizational culture of HCOs in terms of organizational role morality, evaluating whether or how well they have achieved and reinforced the mandates of their roles consistently throughout the organization in all its activities. We also judge HCOs, just as we judge individuals, not merely in terms of role morality, but also from the ideal of moral minimums. In Chapter 2 we articulated some basic moral values, ideals of commonsense morality that are pretty much universally agreed upon as moral minimums for human exchanges and relationships. Some of these values include equal opportunity, mutual respect, avoidance of harms, fairness, respect for basic rights, and keeping one's promises and contracts. These values are often articulated in the mission statements of most HCOs, but more importantly, they serve as external evaluating criteria for judging mission statements, organizational culture, and role practices of HCOs.

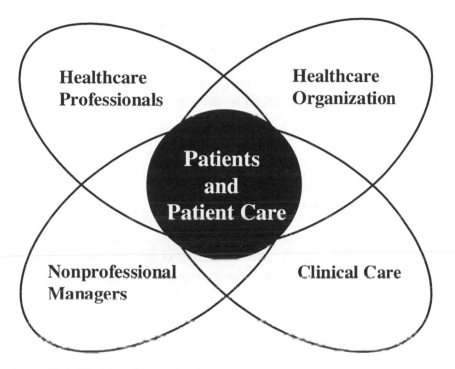

FIGURE 12.1. The idea of an overlapping consensus in HCOs.

Consensus, of course, is not the same as agreement, and consensus on basic mission will not bring agreement in every detail. But consensus on the aims of the organization on how those ends might be prioritized provides a starting point for a dialogue between managers, professionals, payers, and patients. How should this conversation take place? What is needed is a well-articulated organization ethics program that combines the perspectives of clinical ethics, business ethics, and professional ethics as useful analogues for thinking through organization ethics. The purpose of an organization ethics program, as JCAHO states, has to do with the ethical responsibility of an organization to "conduct its business and patient care practices in an honest, decent and proper manner. " Such a program should be able to articulate and apply consistent values in all aspects of the operation of a HCO so that a strong organizational culture and a positive ethical climate can be developed and maintained in all aspects of its operations and with all stakeholders.

Here clinical ethics provides us with a model that has worked well in clinical settings for some time: the institutional ethics committee. Traditionally, healthcare ethics committees have dealt almost exclusively with clinical, health-related dilemmas. But, as we argued in Chapter 9, there is no reason that IECs could not be expanded to represent not merely clinical issues but also professional and economic issues, as well as regulatory policies and challenges. Such a committee could also be in charge of the educational programs at the HCO and from time to time bring in outside consultants to adjudicate various organizational issues and cases. Note that the work of the committee would be primarily to deal with *organizational* issues, not with those that seem solvable by the traditional hospital ethics committees.

As background for the development of a model organization ethics program, Chapters 6 and 7 described the historical development of healthcare organizations and the external social and political climate in which these organizations function today. Then in Chapter 8 through 11 we explored mechanisms for effectively instituting a comprehensive organization ethics program. We discussed how the institution of an organization ethics program can become the sponsor of an all-encompassing positive ethical climate for each HCO. We addressed how this new, more comprehensive perspective can integrate and protect the better-known perspectives of clinical ethics (patient care ethics), business ethics, and professional ethics, while at the same time allowing for a meaningful and effective articulation of each within the context of the rapidly changing healthcare arena. We conclude that a comprehensive organization ethics program that develops and enhances a consistent internal ethical climate through is mission, guidelines, policies, and activities, can and should be of benefit to those responsible for these activities at all levels of the organization.

There are many good reasons why this is the right time to start thinking about organization-wide ethics for HCOs. In Chapters 2 through 5 we presented ethical justification for an organization ethics program. In Chapters 6 and 7 we presented a schematic historical justification for a strong organization ethics program. In those chapters we looked specifically at how shifts in decision-making power altered organizational value priorities. In Chapter 6 we traced the shifts of power and decision-making authority among different groups in the HCO over the last century, culminating in the current situation, described in Chapter 7, where the HCO faces the threat of decision-making authority moving outside the institution entirely.

The current situation is the product of several factors. The price to the patient of the care received has been separated from the cost of that care. The difference between what the patient pays and the actual cost has, for a large portion of the population, been paid by intermediaries: the government, health insurance carriers, or employment-linked health benefits. At the same time, a portion of the population is not in a position to have that difference paid by intermediaries. This uninsured percentage of the population that is unable to receive needed medical care is growing larger.

In the early decades of this century the intermediaries between the patient and the caregivers (healthcare professionals and HCOs) were often religious or charitable foundations using the hospital as their avenue for social responsibility. In the days before medical practice became inextricably intertwined with hospitals, the physician often served as the intermediary between the cost of care and the recipient of the care. As part of his or her individual social responsibility, every doctor in private practice had a roster of patients who were treated at less than cost or for free. After World War II, the major intermediary between the patient and health care, for many of the less prosperous, became the government, through a variety of federal- and state-supported insurance plans for which various categories of people were eligible. As the role of the intermediaries has increased in importance, their nature has changed. Modern participants in the healthcare field (now described as the healthcare industry) include for-profit participants with priorities and obligations that are new. Often they come from areas without the history of social responsibility which characterizes the older players.

All of the contemporary intermediaries have become cost conscious and increasingly reluctant to pay for increases in the costs of health care. One major payer, the government, which supports Medicaid and Medicare plans, is subject to the vagaries of the political process. There is no guarantee that future administrations on either the state or federal level will not shift the provision of health care to the less fortunate further down on their priority list. For employers, healthcare costs are another expense that must be controlled for their own competitive advantage. The businesses that are entering the arena are in the same position.

In contemporary society, the healthcare *organization* is the place where health care is delivered. One of the consequences of recent scientific and technological progress in medicine is to tie the physicians, independent practitioners at the beginning of this century, ever more tightly to the hospital. The relation between physicians and patients is inextricably linked with the fate of hospitals. Healthcare professionals in many specialty areas cannot practice without involving a HCO. Patients cannot get the care they want and expect anywhere else. So the intermediary organizations that are becoming increasingly responsible for the payment for health care of the population cannot do so without the HCO.

No one wishes to see the quality of the medical care delivered in America's HCOs decline. Even the slightest variations in the conditions of care delivery or the quality of care are met with consternation and public outcry. Everyone takes pride in the present standard of medical treatment in this country, the sophisticated technology which facilitates it, and the safe, attentive, and responsible conditions under which it is provided. But maintaining that high quality in the face of the need to restrain costs has become problematic.

The trouble is that the cost-containment and cost-cutting measures have been introduced on the assumption, explicit or tacit, that U.S. health care would continue to be of high quality, that medical science would continue to progress, and that people would get the same care as they had come to expect in the postwar decades when medicine prospered in the United States. There is agreement that cost control is necessary, but little agreement on what measures are appropriate, or even on who should decide what those measures should be. But whoever makes those decisions, it is the HCO that is held responsible for the results.

The HCO faces threats to quality and erosion of confidence. The challenges are to morale, reputation, and financial stability. To meet these challenges the HCO will require a cohesive and integrated internal ethical climate, a consistent commitment to providing excellent care, its major responsibility, and the strong support of its professionals, who remain responsible for the standards of care. We argue that it is only by presenting a united front to external regulators and payers that the HCO can retain control over the decisions which are determining the balance between cost and quality. It is important for morale, reputation, operational excellence, and even for competitive advantage that the HCO take an active role in determining the ethical climate in which health care is delivered. At this historical moment organization ethics represents a route to this end.

Any such organizational initiative will need to meet several conditions. It will need to develop strong reciprocal relations among its internal stakeholders. It must retain traditional values associated with healthcare delivery, despite changing conditions. It should be able to put the HCO in a position to maintain its ethical and quality standards in its relationships with external stakeholders—payers, suppliers, and other contractual partners.

To meet these conditions, we have suggested an organization ethics program that has several characteristics. It integrates clinical, professional, and business ethics in a way that aligns the interests of the organization with its major objectives. It is structured with a modified stakeholder model that presupposes shared responsibility and authority. It develops strong reciprocal relationships between stakeholders, procedural consensus within agreed-upon parameters, and mechanisms for communication, negotiation, and recourse. We have recommended integrating professional ethical standards, including the priority of patient care and the importance of excellent professionally based standards of care, into the mission and values statements, which direct institutional function. We have drawn upon the priorities of clinical ethics, as well as the strengths of its institutional practice, in our recommendations about how the organization ethics process should be instituted.

To be effective, any fully functioning organization ethics program must believe in its stated values and mission, and be committed to putting them into effect in all activities at all levels of the organization. Communication, education, and resolve are key elements in producing a positive ethical climate in an organization, and we have stressed their importance here.

In thinking about ethics in healthcare organizations we have attempted throughout to think about organizations themselves as moral agents, interacting with other moral agents—some individual, some collective. We have emphasized the extent to which, unlike individual moral agents, an HCO is best understood as a dynamic set of processes, structures, and activities. Ethics in organizations plays many of the same roles it plays for individuals: formulating and critiquing goals, determining the appropriateness and moral valence of alternative means to those goals, evaluating habitual behaviors and serving as an internal monitor for the way the institution conducts its activities. Just as responsible individuals must concern themselves with their character, their actions, and their objectives, responsible institutions must do likewise. Organization ethics is formulated as an attempt to meet these goals as well, and to do so in a dynamic, responsive, flexible process.

History illuminates and theory tries to guide, but the real problem facing HCOs today is a practical one. If one wants an organization ethics program (and it is increasingly obvious that every HCO is going to have to have one) what should it look like? How would it be instituted, and how would you tell if it were working? It would be irresponsible to write a book on organization ethics in health care if we were not willing to tackle those practical problems, and we have done so in Chapters 8 through 11.

The organization ethics program we propose is situated at the highest level of the organization. Ideally, it is implemented through a committee composed of members representing all critical areas of the HCO. This model of representation allows the committee to deal in a timely and informed way with all the issues affecting the organizational mission, climate, and operations. It should be able to scrutinize decisions, strategies, policies, or actions that appear to put the institution in ethical conflict with its espoused values as formulated in the mission, code, values statements, or other expressions of ethical standards. In strategizing how such a program might be constructed, we drew on strengths found in clinical, professional, and business ethics, avoiding elements of each that are inappropriate for the more global focus of a healthcare organization ethics program.

This book addresses issues in a new field. We are suggesting a controversial approach, which, if followed, could dramatically affect the current conditions of health care. Our approach is one alternative among many, and we trust that our proposals will provoke a spate of those alternatives in response. Just as we could imagine a "principlist" approach to organization ethics, although we have not chosen to follow that route, we could also have envisaged a more authoritarian approach to the problems we have outlined. Such an approach would differ in some important ways. It might put the organization ethics program in the hands of an individual rather than the committee we recommend. It might subsume the program under one of the organizational units we considered in Chapter 9. As we write, those alternatives and others are being tried out in HCOs across the country.

Although it may have a bright future, organization ethics is in its infancy. We look forward to the responses of the constituencies to whom this book is directed: the managers and nurses, physicians and board members, philosophers and ethics committee members who are engaged with us on the project of helping health care flourish in the future.

Appendix 1

Virginia Bioethics Network
Recommendations for Guidelines on Procedures
and Processes to Address Organization Ethics
in Health Care Organizations

Edward M. Spencer

In 1995 the Virginia Bioethics Network (VBN) adopted "Recommendations for Guidelines on Procedures and Process and Education and Training to Strengthen Bioethics Services in Virginia." This set of guidelines was focused on helping healthcare organizations (HCOs) respond to the needs for ethics services within the organization and surrounding community. The VBN also anticipated that the recommendations could be used as a tool for HCOs to evaluate their ethics services and direct them toward appropriate decisions for improvement of these services. The recommendations also defined certain educational requirements for ethics committee members, ethics consultants, and teachers of introductory and advanced clinical ethics courses.

Since the VBN's action, a number of HCOs, both within Virginia and in other states, have used the recommendations to strengthen and evaluate their individual ethics programs. Many of these HCOs have reported that the recommendations have been valuable in preparing for Joint Commission for Accreditation of Healthcare Organizations (JCAHO) inspections and in addressing issues during the inspections. This positive aspect of the recommendations was not unexpected, since consultation with Paul Schyve, senior vice president, JCAHO, continued throughout their development.

In 1995 JCAHO added a section called "Organization Ethics" to its Standards for Patient Rights and Ethics. This was accomplished without fanfare and with very little notice from the community of HCOs which JCAHO accredits. This change, however, has far-reaching implications for the future operations of HCOs and their internal and external relationships (Including relationships with healthcare professionals and managed-care organizations). Depending on interpretation and implementation, these new standards could well become the framework for assuring ethical oversight of the ever changing healthcare arena for the foreseeable future.

Dr. Schyve has publicly stated on a number of occasions that he believes that the ethics committee in each HCO should be the organizational base for attention to organization ethics. He has challenged the administrations of HCOs to use their ethics committees in this manner and has at the same time challenged ethics committees to rethink and expand their traditional role and services and make necessary changes to respond to this new and important area.

Ethics committees have responded to this challenge in one of two ways: beginning the process of reorganization required by this new mandate by considering the issues of "organization ethics" and developing a strategy to respond, or refusing to become involved at all in organization ethics or asking to be involved only peripherally. VBN believes that the first response is the appropriate one, since it assures that the ethics committee will continue to be a leader in developing and overseeing ethics services within the HCO. This position also assures the HCO board and administration that ethical issues associated with organization ethics will be addressed in an open manner by a committed multidisciplinary group with input from community members, and that ethics processes, which lead to the best in patient care, which assure professional integrity of the practicing clinicians, and which assure that the HCO maintains the highest of ethical standards in its business and management activities, will be developed and maintained.

VBN's board of directors, in its annual meeting in October 1996, voted to develop new guidelines addressing the appropriate response of an HCO's ethics committee to organization ethics issues similar to the recommendations which address the more traditional activities of ethics committees.

The following guidelines have been developed with consultation and input from VBN members and the staff at the University of Virginia's Center for Biomedical Ethics. The guidelines have been revised after input from each of these groups, and the final version has been approved by the VBN board. These new guidelines are only recommendations and are meant to be adopted or rejected piecemeal or in toto by the boards of HCOs. VBN does not claim that these guidelines represent the only or even the best way to respond to the issues of organization ethics. They do, however, represent thoughtful consideration of these issues by VBN member institutions, VBN individual members, and Center staff members with the goal of helping to develop a workable mechanism to address organization ethics issues in each HCO, thereby ensuring ethics oversight of the policies and processes affecting the organizational aspects of the HCO.

We begin with a definition:

> *Organization ethics* consists of a process(es) to address ethical issues associated with the business, financial, and management areas of healthcare organizations, as well as with professional, educational, and contractual relationships affecting the operation of the HCO.

Guideline one: Organization ethics shall be addressed by each HCO's ethics program

VBN believes that the ethics committee is the appropriate body within an HCO to address organization ethics issues for the following reasons:

1. Who better? There is no other established body within healthcare organizations as well prepared to address ethical issues in an open, honest, straightforward manner.
2. By accepting the responsibility for consideration of organization ethics issues, the ethics committee continues as the recognized source for ethics education, consultation, and policy review within the HCO.
3. Although expanding the committee's knowledge base to include the organization ethics arena may be necessary, the process remains essentially the same as that used for consideration of patient care ethics issues.
4. The ethics committee is less likely to be unduly influenced by business, financial, and legal considerations than a group composed of administrators, and/or financial officers, and/or institutional attorneys.
5. Attention to ethical issues in organization ethics is more likely to be accepted by the institution's patients and the community it serves if it is overseen by the ethics committee.

Guideline two: Reorganization of the organization's ethics committee and additional training of ethics committee members shall be undertaken by each HCO so that the ethics program can appropriately respond to organization ethics issues

If organization ethics is to be fully understood by the ethics committee so that it can be fair, objective, and efficient in addressing organization ethics issues, there will, by necessity, need to be changes in the organization and activities of the ethics committee. Following are examples which comprise one workable mechanism for instituting needed changes. Other mechanisms may work as well or better in particular HCOs.

1. Reevaluate the ethics committee's mission statement, policies, and bylaws and change as needed to reflect the expanded scope and activities of the committee in addressing organization ethics issues.
2. Reorganize the ethics committee to include representatives from the business, finance, and management areas of the HCO.
   a. Enlarge committee and expand work to include organization ethics.
   b. Divide the committee into two subcommittees: Patient Care and Organization Ethics. Each subcommittee would have primary responsibility for its particular set of issues with the Patient Care Subcommittee being responsible for the patient care issues traditionally addressed by ethics committees, while the Organization Ethics Subcommittee is responsible for organization ethics issues. Both subcommittees should report to the full committee and any actions or recommendations should be from the full ethics committee after appropriate consideration and discussion.

VBN believes that dividing the committee into two focused subcommittees is the preferred mechanism for reorganization of the committee for most HCOs.

3. Begin an education program focused on organization ethics for committee members. Education should focus on (1) introducing ethics committee members to organization ethics, (2) increasing the committee's knowledge of the business, financial, and management aspects of the HCO, including an introduction to particular ethical issues seen in these areas, (3) a study of conflicts of interest among healthcare professionals, and (4) theoretical and practical issues in business ethics. This may require taking courses at local institutions of higher learning, taking short (one or two-week) intensive courses focused on these issues, contracting with experts to develop and present required education, and discussion concerning these issues among all of the members of the newly formed ethics committee; with the new members from the business, management, and financial areas taking the lead in explaining the ethical principles they use in decision making.

Guideline three: The major functions of the organization ethics activities of the ethics committee shall be to develop or revise an organization code of ethics with attention to the organization's mission statement for guidance; to develop or revise policies which support the mission statement and the code of ethics; to develop an educational program concerning organization ethics issues for board members, clinicians, administrators, finance officers, and community members; and to institute a process for addressing issues and problems which arise in conjunction with organization ethics

1. Develop or review the HCO's code of ethics. The JCAHO now requires that each HCO which it accredits have a code of ethics which addresses at a minimum the following issues: marketing, admission, transfer, discharge, billing practices, providers, payers, and educational institutions. To date, JCAHO has made few specific recommendations as to how the code should address each of these subjects. JCAHO does require that the code be consistent with the mission of the HCO and that, when needed, specific policies be developed to ensure that the code has meaning within the day-to-day operations of the HCO.

   An appropriate first task for the reorganized ethics committee should be review of the code (if one has been developed) with recommendations for change when needed, or the development of the code and supporting policies if this has not been done previously.

2. Develop and institute an educational program focused on organization ethics issues for the committee, the organization's staff, both clinical and nonclinical, and the community which the organization serves.

   The needed education can be accomplished in a number of ways, including lectures from outside experts, lectures from knowledgeable committee members and other staff members, panel discussions, general discussions led by a committee member, case discussions, and a repeatable course developed by the committee. Each committee will decide which of these educational pro-

grams are appropriate for the particular HCO. It is imperative for each ethics committee to begin its educational program as soon as possible and to obtain outside help when needed. (VBN will help its members and others with the development and presentation of educational sessions when needed.)

3. Ethics committees should recognize that certain problems related to organization ethics may occur and a mechanism for addressing these organization ethics "cases" should be developed. The mechanism chosen to address these cases can be similar to the patient care ethics consultation mechanism described in the 1995 recommendations or may take some other form. Whatever approach is selected, a formal process defined by protocol should be developed and instituted; such process to address the issues of access, notice, documentation, and evaluation of the process, as well as education and training of those designated to be responsible for this process.

Guideline four: The organization ethics aspect of the ethics committee shall develop one or more plans for coordination of attention to ethical issues based on the relationships between the HCO and (1) managed care organizations with contractual association, (2) health care professionals, and (3) community organizations with ongoing relationships with the HCO

Relationships and associations (professional, personal, and contractual) among those actively engaged in healthcare delivery are often of primary importance in understanding and resolving ethical problems. In spite of their importance, little attention has been directed toward these issues. VBN believes that the organization ethics activities of the ethics committee should include attention to these important aspects of the ethical climate of the organization.

1. It is appropriate for the ethics committee with an organization ethics function to consider how specific contractual obligations of the HCO do or do not correspond to the stated mission and code of ethics. The ethics committee should have no authority to change these contractual obligations but should be expected to call attention to perceived deviations from the mission and code within the organization.
2. It is appropriate for an ethics committee with an organization ethics function to offer assistance to healthcare professionals when problems occur based on conflicts between professional obligations and obligations imposed by administrative and regulatory structures. The ethics committee should not, however, be involved in strictly professional issues.
3. The ethics committee with an organization ethics function should recognize as part of its obligation enhancement of disclosure and communication between the HCO and (1) its employees, (2) its professional staff, (3) its contractual partners, and (4) most importantly, the community it serves.

Approved October 25, 1997

Appendix 2

Towards a Pragmatic Method for Assessing Moral Problems

Donald W. Light

Framing the problem

1. *Whose problem is it anyway?*
   Who is defining something as a "problem" and what are the frameworks being used to define it as a problem? What interests or stakes do the defining party and the parties affected have?
2. *Who makes up the moral community in which the problem is said to exist?*
   What is the character of that community? What are its values? How does it relate to the moral community of the patient and other significant parties?
3. *How has the problem developed over its full history?*
   What processes of legitimization and institutionalization have taken place?
4. *How have decisions by institutional powers, like medical, economic, political, and professional organizations, shaped the nature of the problem and the range of options available?*
   How is the problem sociologically embedded? In what ways have economic, institutional, and professional priorities created, exacerbated, or facilitated the problem and possible solutions?
5. *How does the political economy of the situation or program affect the issue and its possible resolutions?*
   Who is sponsoring the program and what are their interests? Who established the rules or program? Were and are those affected consulted? Were and are they fully informed about the program and its effects on them?

Parsing the problem

6. *What are the issues or dilemmas that make up the problem?*
   Which parties are trying to do, or resist? What are their fears, hopes, or intentions? What are the dynamics of rule breaking, deviance, and legitimacy going on?
7. *What are the technical aspects of the problem?*
   How do technical procedures, devices, or agents affect how the problem is defined and what options are possible? How does the scientific or techno-

logical framing of the problem affect its perception? What are the roles of experts and expertise?

8. *What harms are being alleged, and by whom?*
What kinds of harms are they? How imminent or latent are they? What are the costs of the alleged harms, and to which parties?

9. *What are the social and cultural relationships and context?*
Look at roles, role sets, role conflicts, statuses, norms, traditions, and taboos.

10. *How much choice do the key parties have and how do they exercise it?*
Consider the continuum of restraints on choice, including habits, routines, rituals, obsessions, prejudices, addictions, and genetics.

11. *What are the options? How might the problem be resolved in win-win ways?*
What values, principles, or priorities might most appropriately be invoked, now that the full institutional, historical, hierarchical, and relational nature of the situations is known? At what level should solutions be addressed?

12. *Whose interests are you serving?*
Who invited you? Who is paying you? On whom do you depend for your current and future work? Are you attending fully to the patient and empowering her or him to give voice to her or his concerns and preferences? If the problem or its solutions point to prejudices, institutional practices, or forms of economic or political oppression, are you addressing these?

January 1999

Appendix 3

A Decision Process:
A Framework for Moral Reasoning

- What are the facts?
- What is the background, and external social/political/legal climate in which this organizational issue is imbedded?
- What is the organization's mission and organizational culture in this case?
- What are the ethical issues?
    From the manager's perspective?
    From the professional's perspective?
    From the clinical and patient perspective?
    From the organization's perspective?
- Who are the primary stakeholders?
- What are the viable alternatives?
- How do you defend those alternatives?
    What core values are at stake?
    Who is harmed? Who benefits?
    What rights are at stake?
    Can you defend this action publicly?
    What kind of precedent does it set?
- What are the practical constraints?
- What is the best choice, or least harmful, all things considered?
- What is the implementation plan for the alternative that you have chosen?

Adapted with modifications from the Arthur Andersen Program in Business Ethics' Seven Step Model for Moral Reasoning. © 1991 Arthur Andersen & Co. C.I.E.

Appendix 4

Codes of Ethics

The American Medical Association: Principles of Medical Ethics

The medical profession has long subscribed to a body of ethical statements developed primarily for the benefit of the patient. As a member of this profession, a physician must recognize responsibility not only to patients, but also to society, to other health professionals, and to self. The following principles adopted by the American Medical Association are not laws, but standards of conduct which define the essentials of honorable behavior for the physician.

    I. A physician shall be dedicated to providing competent medical service with compassion and respect for human dignity.

    II. A physician shall deal honestly with patients and colleagues, and strive to expose those physicians deficient in character or competence, or who engage in fraud or deception.

    III. A physician shall respect the law and also recognize a responsibility to seek changes in those requirements which are contrary to the best interests of the patient.

    IV. A physician shall respect the rights of patients, or colleagues, and of other health professionals, and shall safeguard patient confidences within the constraints of the law.

    V. A physician shall continue to study, apply, and advance scientific knowledge, make relevant information available to patients, colleagues, and the public, obtain consultation, and use the talents of other health professionals when indicated.

    VI. A physician shall, in the provision of appropriate patient care, except in emergencies, be free to choose whom to serve, with whom to associate, and the environment in which to provide medical services.

    VII. A physician shall recognize a responsibility to participate in activities contributing to an improved community.

The American Nurses Association: Code for Nurses

    1. The nurse provides services with respect for human dignity and the uniqueness of the client unrestricted by considerations of social or economic status, personal attributes, or the nature of health problems.

2. The nurse safeguards the client's right to privacy by judiciously protecting information of a confidential nature.
3. The nurse acts to safeguard the client and the public when health care and safety are affected by the incompetent, unethical, or illegal practice of any person.
4. The nurse assumes responsibility and accountability for individual nursing judgements and actions.
5. The nurse maintains competence in nursing.
6. The nurse exercises informed judgement and uses individual competence and qualifications as criteria in seeking consultation, accepting responsibilities, and delegating nursing activities to others.
7. The nurse participates in activities that contribute to the ongoing development of the profession's body of knowledge.
8. The nurse participates in the profession's efforts to implement and improve standards of nursing.
9. The nurse participates in the profession's efforts to establish and maintain conditions of employment conducive to high quality nursing care.
10. The nurse participates in the profession's effort to protect the public from misinformation and misrepresentation and to maintain the integrity of nursing.
11. The nurse collaborates with members of the health professions and other citizens in promoting community and national efforts to meet the health needs of the public.

Code of Ethics of the American College of Healthcare Executives, as amended by the Council of Regents at its annual meeting on August 22, 1995

Preface

The Code of Ethics is administered by the Ethics Committee, which is appointed by the Board of Governors upon nomination by the Chairman. It is composed of at least nine Fellows of the College, each of whom serves a three-year term on a staggered basis, with three members retiring each year.

The Ethics Committee shall:

- Review and evaluate annually the Code of Ethics, and make any necessary recommendations for updating the Code.
- Review and recommend action to the Board of Governors on allegations brought forth regarding breaches of the Code of Ethics.
- Develop ethical policy statements to serve as guidelines of ethical conduct for healthcare executives and their professional relationships.
- Prepare an annual report of observations, accomplishments, and recommendations to the Board of Governors, and such other periodic reports as required.

The Ethics Committee invokes the Code of Ethics under authority of the ACHE Bylaws, Article II, Membership, Section 6, Resignation and Termination of Membership; Transfer to Inactive Status, subsection (b), as follows:

> Membership may be terminated or rendered inactive by action of the Board of Governors as a result of violation of the Code of Ethics; nonconformity with the Bylaws or Regulations Governing Admission, Advancement, Recertification, and Reappointment; conviction of a felony; or conviction of a crime of moral turpitude or a crime relating to the healthcare management profession. No such termination of membership or imposition of inactive status shall be affected without affording a reasonable opportunity for the member to consider the charges and to appear in his or her own defense before the Board of Governors or its designated hearing committee, as outlined in the "Grievance Procedure," Appendix I of the College's Code of Ethics.

Preamble

The purpose of the Code of Ethics of the American College of Healthcare Executives is to serve as a guide to conduct its members. It contains standards of ethical behavior for healthcare executives in their professional relationships. These relationships include members of the healthcare executive's organization and other organizations. Also included are patients or others served, colleagues, the community, and society as a whole. The Code of Ethics also incorporates standards of ethical behavior governing personal behavior, particularly when that conduct directly relates to the role and identity of the healthcare executive.

The fundamental objectives of the healthcare management profession are to enhance overall quality of life, dignity, and well-being of every individual needing healthcare services; and to create a more equitable, accessible, effective, and efficient healthcare system.

In fulfilling their commitments and obligations to patients or others served, healthcare executives function as moral advocates. Since every management decision affects the health and well-being of both individuals and communities, healthcare executives must carefully evaluate the possible outcomes of their decisions. In organizations that deliver healthcare services, they must work to safeguard and foster rights, interests, and prerogatives of patients or others served. The role of moral advocate requires that healthcare executives speak out and take actions necessary to promote such rights, interests, and prerogatives if they are threatened.

I. The healthcare executive's responsibilites to the profession of healthcare management

The healthcare executive shall:

A. Uphold the values, ethics and mission of the healthcare management profession;

B. Conduct all personal and professional activities with honesty, integrity, repect, fairness, and good faith in a manner that will reflect well upon the profession;

C. Comply with all laws pertaining to healthcare management in the jurisdictions in which the healthcare executive is located, or conducts professional activities;

D. Maintain competence and proficiency in healthcare management by implementing a personal program of assessment and continuing professional education;

E. Avoid the exploitation of professional relationships for personal gain;

F. Use this Code to further the interests of the profession and not for selfish reasons;

G. Respect professional confidences;

H. Enhance the dignity and image of the healthcare management profession through positive public information programs; and

I. Refrain from participating in any activity that demeans the credibility and dignity of the healthcare management profession.

II. The healthcare executive's responsibilities to patients or others served, to the organization, and to employees

A. Responsibilities to patients or others served

The healthcare executive shall, within the scope of his or her authority:

1. Work to ensure the existence of a process to evaluate the quality of care or service rendered;

2. Avoid practicing or facilitating discrimination and institute safeguards to prevent discriminatory organizational practices;

3. Work to ensure the existence of a process that will advise patients or others served of the rights, opportunities, responsibilities, and risks regarding available healthcare services;

4. Work to provide a process that ensures the autonomy and self-determination of patients or others served; and

5. Work to ensure the existence of procedures that will safeguard the confidentiality and privacy of patients or others served.

B. Responsibilities to the organization

The healthcare executive shall, within the scope of his or her authority:

1. Provide healthcare services consistent with available resources and work to ensure the existence of a resource allocation process that considers ethical ramifications;

2. Conduct both competitive and cooperative activities in ways that improve community healthcare services;

3. Lead the organization in the use and improvement of standards of management and sound business practices;
4. Respect the customs and practices of patients or others served, consistent with the organization's philosophy; and
5. Be truthful in all forms of professional and organizational communication, and avoid disseminating information that is false, misleading, or deceptive.

C. Responsibilities to employees

Healthcare executives have an ethical and professional obligation to employees of the organizations they manage that encompass but are not limited to:

1. Working to create a working environment conducive for underscoring employee ethical conduct and behavior.
2. Working to ensure that individuals may freely express ethical concerns and providing mechanisms for discussing and addressing such concerns.
3. Working to ensure a working environment that is free from harassment, sexual and other, coercion of any kind, especially to perform illegal or unethical acts; and discrimination on the basis of race, creed, color, sex, ethnic origin, age, or disability.
4. Working to ensure a working environment that is conducive to proper utilization of employees' skills and abilities.
5. Paying particular attention to the employee's work environment and job safety.
6. Working to establish appropriate grievance and appeals mechanisms.

III. Conflicts of Interest

A conflict of interest may be only a matter of degree, but exists when the healthcare executive:

A. Acts to benefit directly or indirectly by using authority or inside information, or allows a friend, relative, or associate to benefit from such authority or information.
B. Uses authority or information to make a decision to intentionally affect the organization in an adverse manner.

The healthcare executive shall:

A. Conduct all personal and professional relationships in such a way that all those affected are assured that management decisions are made in the best interests of the organization and the individuals served by it;
B. Disclose to the appropriate authority any direct or indirect financial or personal interests that pose potential or actual conflicts of interest;

C. Accept no gifts or benefits offered with the express or implied expectation of influencing a management decision; and
D. Inform the appropriate authority and other involved parties of potential or actual conflicts of interest related to appointments or elections to boards or committees inside or outside the healthcare executive's organization.

IV. The healthcare executive's responsibilities to community and society

The healthcare executive shall:

A. Work to identify and meet the healthcare needs of the community;
B. Work to ensure that all people have reasonable access to healthcare services;
C. Participate in public dialogue on healthcare policy issues and advocate solutions that will improve health status and promote quality healthcare;
D. Consider the short-term and long-term impact of management decisions on both the community and on society; and
E. Provide prospective consumers with adequate and accurate information, enabling them to make enlightened judgements and decisions regarding services.

V. The healthcare executive's responsibility to report violations of the code

A member of the College who has reasonable grounds to believe that another member has violated this Code has a duty to communicate such facts to the Ethics Committee.

Appendix 5

The Rise, Fall, and Reemergence of the Nursing Home: Important Lessons to Be Learned

"It has been said that the moral heart of a society can be judged by how well it provides for those at the dawn of life, those in the shadows of life, and those in the twilight of life. Nursing homes are places of lengthening shadows at twilight. By and large they are the last refuge in our society's broader system—if such a tattered, patchwork arrangement of overlapping and conflicting programs can be called that—of social support and provision for the elderly, the frail, and those with chronic illness and disability." (Collopy, Boyle & Jennings, 1991, p. 1)

With the above paragraph the special report on nursing home ethics published in the Hastings Center Report in 1991 was introduced. This report was the result of a two year study supported by the Pew Memorial Trust. One reason for this study was a belief that our society has not truly worked out a moral vision of the nursing home and what it should be. There are many reasons for this but, just as with the hospital and its ethical climate, the history of the development of nursing homes has much to do with its present position and moral vision.

In many ways the nursing home is a direct descendent of the almshouse. Prior to the twentieth century, relatives or friends cared for the poor elderly, frail, and those with disabilities. When this support system was unavailable, they were relegated to the almshouse, or the poorhouse, as it was sometimes called. Nineteenth-century social morality looked upon poverty and disability as signs of lack of individual moral worth, and so the fact that the almshouse was unpleasant and sometimes harsh was to some extent a way to convince citizens to avoid it at all costs. At the beginning of the twentieth century a few churches and benevolent community organizations began to sponsor old-age homes, but the county or city poorhouse continued to be a fact of life until after the Second World War. During the first half of the twentieth century the poorhouse became a common site for the destitute elderly to spend the final days of their lives.

During the Great Depression of the 1930s there was a tremendous increase in numbers of dependent elderly who had no other resources for care. The passage of the Social Security Act is believed by many to have given the elderly greater resources to determine their own destiny in the waning years of their life, even when there were no family members or friends to offer lodging and food.

Social Security did not directly fund nursing home care but it did put a certain degree of financial power in the hands of the elderly and allowed many to escape public dependency and relegation to the poorhouse. Increased funding of individual elderly citizens under Social Security supported the growth of for-profit nursing homes for the elderly and led to the long-awaited demise of the poorhouse. The precedent set by the Hill-Burton Act, which supported the building of a large number of hospital beds, was expanded to include nonprofit nursing homes soon after its passage and, ultimately, partially subsidized proprietary nursing homes as well.

As post–World War II hospitals became more and more technologically driven and medical specialist oriented, the rapidly developing nursing home industry was left to fulfill the need for long-term care of the elderly (and others who were disabled). As Collopy noted, "By the 1960s, then, the nursing home had emerged as the clearly recognized institutional setting for the long-term care of the elderly" (p. 4).

The major financial boon to the development of nursing homes was Medicaid, which at present covers over 50 percent of nursing home costs. In the 1960s as institutions for care of mental patients were closed, these patients frequently ended up in nursing homes with payment for their care coming from Medicaid or other government-sponsored programs.

By the late 1960s and early '70s there were numerous revelations of illegal and unethical practices in the nursing home industry. There were repeated stories in the press of abuse of nursing home residents, of clearly substandard care, of negligence, and most particularly of extortion, fraud, and embezzlement. To correct these almost universal problems, federal and state governments instituted a number of reforms and, most important, instituted regulations addressing all aspects of nursing home operation. This industry is at present so regulated that there is little freedom to institute even helpful innovations unless fully approved by the regulators. The bureaucratic requirements for change are so onerous that even the most dedicated nursing home operator and administrator often do not even attempt to get permission for changes they are certain would be beneficial for their residents. Nursing homes today are safe but often sterile places.

At present there are over 16,000 nursing homes in the United States (about 66 percent for-profit and often managed as chains, 26 percent nonprofit, and 7 percent government operated). Costs in 1995 for the average resident in a nursing home were over $46,000 a year. Just over 35 percent of the total costs are paid from direct payments from the residents, about 60 percent from government funds (54 percent Medicaid and 6 percent Medicare), and the rest from private insurance and other income sources. Because of the costs, most nursing home residents begin their stints in nursing homes by paying full costs but soon find that they have used all available resources and must then rely on Medicaid assistance for the funding of their nursing home care. This "spending down" commonly occurs during the first year of nursing home residency, meaning that residents who stay in a nursing home for more than one year are more likely to be recipients of government largess for their care (just as it was with the poorhouse in earlier days). Recent federal legislation allows an elderly Medicaid recipient to keep his family home even while on Medicaid.

The image of the nursing home continues to be a problem, since it often conjures up earlier problems with neglect and abandonment and the image of the residents as a dependent, socially undesirable group. Few elders choose nursing home care even when it is obvious that it would be the most appropriate care for them at this time of their life. The social stigma of the poorhouse remains and the stigma of the residents as less desirable citizens also still remains. Families which must deal with the difficulty and pain of "institutionalizing" one of their elderly loved ones face these stigmas as well as the guilt associated with the often mistaken belief that they are being unfair and are not fulfilling their familial obligations. Family members and others may look upon nursing home admission as a form of abandonment and, no matter how necessary, admission of a family member to a nursing home is seldom easy.

On the brighter side, many (probably most) nursing homes today are looking internally at their institutions and their activities in terms of their ethical climate. They are clarifying the differences between nursing homes and acute-care hospitals and teaching their employees, their residents, and their communities about these differences and what they mean for the nursing home and its residents. The acute-care hospital admits the patient with hopes for a cure, assuming decision-making capacity, with the expectation that any disability will be temporary. Any necessary restrictions of freedom are assumed to be acceptable because of their temporary nature. For the nursing home resident, the facility is his home. Capacity may be present or absent and may change, and disabilities are not likely to be cured, but the resident needs help in coping with the disability. Any restrictions of freedom need to be clearly stated at the time of admission and most can be negotiated.

The individual autonomy of the nursing home resident should probably not be considered the absolute mechanism for assuring self-determination. Instead we need to support the development of a concept of community-based autonomy, which is not separate from the social and personal (particularly mental capacity). Care in a nursing home involves everyday living. It is not external and temporary but is the fabric of the resident's life now and for the future. Issues of personal control and the limitations inherent in the setting need to be considered within the context of ongoing incremental flow of acceptance and refusal, negotiation and trial, and acquiescence and noncooperation (Collopy, Boyle & Jennings, 1991, p. 9).

As can be understood from the foregoing brief description, the ethical climate and its road to development in a nursing home is likely to be quite different from the ethical climate of an acute-care HCO. An ethical nursing home must consider a resident's needs and desires, but within the constraints of maintaining a safe and pleasant environment for all the residents. To remain in operation it must attend to a myriad of regulations, so burdensome as to sometimes seem to be the only thing that gets done. There are always problems with maintaining individual privacy and addressing issues such as noise, interpersonal relationships among residents (and staff), and care for the mentally and physically incapacitated.

The amount of control that any individual resident may exercise at any given time is a function of many variables, many of which are beyond the control of the individual resident.

The values underlying nursing home care are often similar in different nursing homes. Developing and maintaining a safe and pleasant environment for the residents; attending to medical and day-to-day living needs, supporting an environment which feels to the constituents like a community, and doing this for a reasonable fee. Honesty, beneficence, and disclosure of conflicts affecting residents are all laudable virtues for nursing home staffs and are frequently mentioned in values and mission statements. The ethical climate of the nursing home is in reality determined by the interactions among several groups ("stakeholders" in business ethics parlance) including owners, administrators, staff and employees, and, most important, the residents and their families.

The nursing home in many cases supports the ideal we are advocating in this book by considering the ethical stance of each of these groups and making an attempt at integrating them into a consistent ethical climate. Its major problem to date has been its lack of ability to develop a consistent and effective mechanism to develop and maintain its ethical climate in the face of intrusive regulation and narrow financial margins. What this has meant is that most nursing homes do not have the time or do not make the effort to develop and maintain their ethical climate. To us, it seems time to institute some degree of regulatory relief. This may be necessary before nursing homes can spare the effort to develop and maintain such an ethical climate.

References

Abrams, F. (1997). Do We Still Need Doctors? Book Review of J. Lantos. *Journal of the American Medical Association*, 278(13). P. 1123.

American College of Healthcare Executives. (1998). *Code of Ethics. http://www.ache.org*

American College of Healthcare Executives. Available: *http://ache.org/policy/pps2.html*

American College of Physicians. (1998). *Ethics Manual*. (4th. ed.), Philadelphia, PA: ACP.

American Hospital Association. (1997). Case Statement. *AHA's Organization Ethics Initiative*. Chicago: AHA, pp. 1–4.

American Medical Association Council on Ethical and Judicial Affairs. (1996). *Code of Medical Ethics, Current Opinions and Annotations*. Chicago: American Medical Association.

Andre, J. (1991). Role Morality as a Complex Instance of Ordinary Morality. *American Philosophical Quarterly*, 28. Pp. 73–80.

———. (1998). Personal Communication.

Appleby, C. (1996). True Values. While Ethical Decision Making and Managed Care Aren't Mutually Exclusive, Executives Are Struggling to Find a Common Denominator. *Hospitals and Health Networks*, 70(13). Pp. 20–22, 26.

Arendt, H. (1963). *Eichmann in Jerusalem*. New York: Viking Press.

Association of American Medical Colleges. (1993). *Guidelines for Dealing with Faculty Conflicts of Commitment and Conflicts of Interest in Research*. Washington, DC: Association of American Medical Colleges.

Barber, B. (1988). Professions and Emerging Professions. Reprinted in J. Callahan, *Ethical Issues in Professional Life*. New York. Oxford University Press.

Bayles, M. (1981). *Professional Ethics*. Belmont, CA: Wadsworth Publishing.

Beauchamp, T. L., & Childress, J. F. (1994). *Principles of Biomedical Ethics*. (4th. ed.). New York: Oxford University Press.

Bedau, H. (1992). Applied Ethics. *Encyclopedia of Ethics*. Lawrence Becker (Ed.). New York: Garland Publishers, pp. 49–52.

The Belmont Report: Ethical Principles and Guidelines for the Protection of Human Subjects of Research. (1978). Washington, DC: U.S. Government Printing Office DHEW Pub. No. (OS) 78-0012.

Benner, P. (1990). The Moral Dimensions of Caring. In J. Stevenson & T. Tripp-Reimer (Eds.), *Knowledge about Care and Caring: State of the Art and Future Developments*. Kansas City: American Academy of Nursing, pp. 5–17.

———. (1991). The Role of Experience, Narrative, and Community in Skilled Ethical Comportment. *Advances in Nursing Science*, 14. Pp. 1–21.

Bentham, J. (1789; 1948). *An Introduction to the Principles of Morals and Legislation*. New York: Hafner Publishing Company.

Blendon, R., et al. (1998). Understanding the Managed Care Backlash. *Health Affairs*, 17(1). Pp. 80–93.

Bowden, P. (1997). *Caring: Gender-Sensitive Ethics*. London: Routledge.

Bowie, N. (1999). *Kantian Capitalism.* Boston: Blackwell Publishers.

Brodie, M., Brady, L., & Altman, D. (1998). Media Coverage of Managed Care: Is There a Negative Bias? *Health Affairs,* 17(1). Pp. 9–34.

Brody, Baruch. (1988). *Life and Death Decision Making.* Oxford: Oxford University Press.

Buchanan, A. (1996). Toward a Theory of the Ethics of Bureaucratic Organizations. *Business Ethics Quarterly.* Pp. 419–440.

Callahan, D. (1995). Bioethics. In W. T. Reich (Ed.), *Encyclopedia of Bioethics.* (Revised ed.). New York: Macmillan Library Reference, pp. 247–256.

Carson, P., Carson, K., & Roe, C. (1995). *Management of Healthcare Organizations.* Cincinnati: South-Western College Publishing.

Casarett, D. J., Frona, D., & Lantos, J. (1998). Experts in Ethics? The Authority of the Clinical Ethicist. *Hastings Center Report,* 28(6). Pp. 6–11.

Chambliss, D. F. (1996). *Beyond Caring: Hospitals, Nurses and the Social Organization of Ethics.* Chicago: University of Chicago Press.

Christensen, K. T. (1996). Ethically Important Distinctions among Managed Care Organizations. *Journal of Law, Medicine & Ethics,* 23. Pp. 223–229.

Clancy, C. (1995). Managed Care: Jekyll or Hyde? *Journal of the American Medical Association,* 273(4). Pp. 338–339.

Clouser, K. D., & Gert, B. (1990). A Critique of Principlism. *Journal of Medicine and Philosophy,* 15(2). Pp. 219–236.

Colby, D. C. (1997) Doctors and Their Discontents. *Health Affairs,* 6(7), pp. 112–114.

Collins, J., & Porras, J. (1994). *Built to Last: Successful Habits of Visionary Companies.* New York: HarperCollins Publishers.

Collopy, B., Boyle, P., & Jennings, B. (1991). New Directions in Nursing Home Ethics. *Hastings Center Report,* 21(2). Special Supplement. B. J. Crigger (Ed.).

Cooper, M. C. (1990). Reconceptualizing Nursing Ethics. *Scholarly Inquiry for Nursing Practice,* 4(3). Pp. 209–221.

Council of Medical Specialty Societies. (1998). *Consensus Statement on the Ethic of Medicine.* Lake Bluff, IL: Council of Medical Specialty Societies, p. 2.

Council Report. (1995). Ethical Issues in Managed Care. *Journal of American Medical Association,* 273. Pp. 330–335.

Crane, D. (1997). *The Sanctity of Social Life: Physicians Treatment of Critically Ill Patients.* New Brunswick, NJ: Transaction Books.

Dalton, D., Metzger, M., & Hill, J. (1994). U.S. Sentencing Commission Guidelines: A Wake-Up Call for Corporate America. In T. Donaldson & P. Werhane (Eds.), *Ethical Issues in Business.* Upper Saddle River, NJ: Prentice-Hall, pp. 331–336.

Darr, K. (1997). *Ethics in Health Services Management.* (3rd. ed.). Baltimore: Health Professions Press, p. 52.

Deming, W. E. (1981–1982). Improvement of Quality and Productivity through Action by Management. *National Productivity Review,* 1(1). Pp. 12–22.

Donaldson, T., & Dunfee, T. (1994). Toward a Unified Conception of Business Ethics: Integrative Social Contracts Theory. *Academy of Management Review* 18(2). Pp. 22–284.

———. (1995). Integrative Social Contracts Theory: A Communitarian Conception of Economic Ethics. *Economics and Philosophy,* 11. Pp. 85–112.

Donaldson, T., & Preston, L. (1995). The Stakeholder Theory of the Corporation: Concepts, Evidence, and Implications. *Academy of Management Review,* 20. Pp. 65–91.

Downie, R. S. (1971). *Roles and Values.* London: Methuen.

Drane, J. F. (1994). *Clinical Bioethics: Theory and Practice in Medical-Ethical Decision Making.* Kansas City: Sheed and Ward.

Eddy, D. (1998). Performance Measurement: Problems and Solutions. *Health Affairs*, 17(4). Pp. 7–15.

Emanuel, E. J. (1995). Preserving the Physician-Patient Relationship in the Era of Managed Care. *Journal of American Medical Association*, 273(4). Pp. 323–329.

Emanuel, E. J., & Emanuel, L. L. (1996). What Is Accountability in Health Care? *Annals of Internal Medicine*, 124. Pp. 229–239.

Emmet, D. (1966). *Rules, Roles and Relation.* New York: St. Martin's Press.

Evan, W., & Freeman, R. E. (1996). A Stakeholder Theory of the Modern Corporation: Kantian Capitalism. In T. Donaldson & P. Werhane (Eds.), *Ethical Issues in Business* (5th ed.). Upper Saddle River, NJ: Prentice-Hall. Pp. 311–315.

Federal Sentencing Guidelines. (1995a). Available: http://www.ussc.gov/guide/ch8web.htm.
———. (1995b). Authority. Available: http://www.ussc.gov/guide/ch1web.htm.
———. (1995c). Historical Note. Available: http://www.ussc.gov/guide/ch8web.htm.

Flanagan, L. (1976). *One Strong Voice: The Story of the American Nurses' Association.* Kansas City: American Nurses' Association.

Fletcher, J., & Brody, H. (1995). Clinical Ethics. In W. T. Reich (Ed.), *Encyclopedia of Bioethics.* (Revised ed.). New York: Macmillan Library Reference, pp. 399–404.

Fletcher, J., Lombardo, P. A., Marshall, M. F., & Miller, F. G. (Eds.). (1997). *Introduction to Clinical Ethics.* (2nd ed.). Frederick, MD: University Publishing Group.

Forehand, B., Gilmer, B. (1964). Environmental Variation in Studies of Organization Behavior. *Psychological Bulletin*, 62. Pp. 361–382.

Fox, E. (1996). Concepts in Evaluation Applied to Ethics Consultation Research. *Journal of Clinical Ethics*, 7(2). Pp.116–121.

Fox, E. & Arnold, R. (1996,). Evaluating Outcomes in Ethics Consultation Research. *Journal of Clinical Ethics,* 7(2). Pp.127–138.

Francis, J. (1997). The Cost Management Imperative. In W. Lerner (Ed.), *Anatomy of a Merger: BJC Health System.* Chicago: Health Administration Press FACHE, p. 231.

Freeman R. E. (1999). Stakeholder Theory and the Modern Corporation. Reprinted in T. Donaldson and P. H. Werhane (Eds.), *Ethical Issues in Business.* (6th. ed.). Upper Saddle River, NJ: Prentice-Hall, pp. 247–257.
———. (1984). *Strategic Management: A Stakeholder Approach.* Boston: Pitman Publishing.
———. (1994). The Politics of Stakeholder Theory: Some Future Directions. *Business Ethics Quarterly*, 4. Pp. 409–422.

French, P. (1979). The Corporation as a Moral Person. *American Philosophical Quarterly*, 16. Pp. 207–215.

Friedman, M. (1970). The Social Responsibility of Business Is to Increase its Profits. *New York Times Magazine*, September 1. Pp. 122–126.
———. (1987). Care and Context in Moral Reasoning. In E. F. Kittay & D. T. Meyers (Eds.), *Women and Moral Theory.* Totowa, NJ: Rowman and Littlefield, pp. 190–204.

FTC Antitrust Actions in Health Care Services. (1999). Available: http://www.ftc.gov/bc/atahcsvs.htm.

Fuchs, V. R., & Garber, A. M. (1990). The New Technology Assessment. *New England Journal of Medicine*, 323(10). Pp. 673–677.

Gadow, S. (1988). Covenant without Cure: Letting Go and Holding On in Chronic Illness. In J. Watson & M. Ray (Eds.), *The Ethics of Care and the Ethics of Cure: Synthesis in Chronicity.* New York: National League of Nursing.

Garrison, R., & Noreen, E. (1997). *Managerial Accounting.* (8th. ed.). Boston: Irwin McGraw-Hill, pp. 200–202.

Goldman, A. (1980). *The Moral Foundations of Professional Ethics*. Totowa, NJ: Rowman and Littlefield.

Goldman, F. (1948). *Voluntary Medical Care Insurance in the United States*. New York, NY: Columbia Press, p. 59.

Goldsmith, J. (1998). Columbia/HCA: A Failure of Leadership. *Health Affairs*, 17(2). Pp. 27–39.

Goodpaster, K. (1982). Morality and Organizations. In T. Donaldson & P. Werhane (Eds.), *Ethical Issues in Business*. (2nd. ed.). Englewood Cliffs, NJ: Prentice Hall, pp. 137–145.

———. (1984). The Concept of Corporate Responsibility. In T. Regan (Ed.), *Just Business*. New York: Random House, pp. 292–323.

———. (1992). Business Ethics. In L. Becker (Ed.), *Encyclopedia of Ethics*. New York: Garland Publishers, pp. 111–115.

Gray, B. H. (1997). Conversion of HMOs and Hospitals: What's at Stake? *Health Affairs*, 16(2). Pp. 29–47.

Greenlick, M. R., Freeborn, D. K., & Pope, C. R. (1988). Background. In M. R. Greenlick, D. K. Freeborn, & C. R. Pope (Eds.), *Healthcare Research in an HMO*. Baltimore, MD: The Johns Hopkins University Press.

HCFA Statistics: Expentitures. *HCFA Statistics 1996*. Pp. 1–14. Online. 6 June 1997. Available http://www.hcfa.gov/stats/stats.htm.

Hardimon, M. (1994). Role Obligations. *Journal of Philosophy*, 91. Pp. 333–363.

Hausman, D. M., & McPherson, M. S. (1996). *Economic Analysis and Moral Philosophy*. Cambridge: Cambridge University Press.

HFMA Express News, 25 April 1997. Available: http://www.hma.com/dojstres.html.

HFMA Press Release, 17 November 1997. Available: http://www.hfma.org/about/nov17p.htm.

Healthcare Management Advisors. (1997). Model Compliance Plan for Clinical Labs. *HFMA Express News*, February 28. Available: http://www.hma.com/complan.html.

Hekman, S. J. (1995). *Moral Voices, Moral Selves*. Cambridge: Polity Press.

Holleman, W. L., Edwards, D. C., & Matson, C. C. (1994). Obligations of Physicians to Patients and Third Party Payers. *Journal of Clinical Ethics*, 5(2). Pp. 113–120.

Hollis, S. (1997). Conversion of Non-Profit Hospitals. *Health Affairs*, 16(2). Pp. 132–143.

Http://www.ftc.gov/reports/hlth3s.htm#1.

Http://www.st-marys.org/mission.html.

Http://www.nchc.org.

Http://www.wnet.org/archive/mhc/Info/Glossary/Glossary.htm1#HMO).

Http://managed care mag.com/archiveMC/9705/9795./erisa.shtml.

Http://www.osha.gov/cgi-bin/sic/sicser?6324.

Hughes, E. C. (1963). Professions. Reprinted in J. Callahan, *Ethical Issues in Professional Life*. (1998). New York: Oxford University Press.

Hume, D. (1909). *Dialogues Concerning Natural Religion*. London: Longmans & Green.

Husted, G. L., & Husted, J. H. (1991). *Ethical Decision-Making in Nursing*. St. Louis: Mosby-Yearbook, pp. 27–38.

Iglehart, J. K. (1994). Physicians and the Growth of Managed Care. *New England Journal of Medicine*, 327. Pp. 1167–1171.

Isaacs, S., Beatrice, D., & Carr, W. (1997). Health Care Conversion Foundations: A Status Report. *Health Affairs*, 16(6). Pp. 228–236.

Jacques, E. (1951). *The Changing Culture of a Factory*. New York: Dryden Press.

Joint Commission for Accreditation of Healthcare Organizations. (1992). Patient Rights. *1992 Accreditation Manual for Hospitals.* Chicago, IL: JCAHO, pp. 103–105.

———. (1995). Patient Rights and Organization Ethics. *Comprehensive Manual for Hospitals.* Chicago, IL: JCAHO, pp. 95–96.

———. (1996). Patient Rights and Organizational Ethics: Standards for Organizational Ethics. *1996 Comprehensive Manual for Hospitals.* Chicago, IL: JCAHO, pp. 95–97.

———. (1997). Patient Rights and Organization Ethics. *1997 Comprehensive Accreditation Manual for Hospitals: The Official Handbook.* Chicago, IL: JCAHO, RI-1–RI-32.

Jones, D. (1997). Putting Patients First: A Philosophy in Practice. *Health Affairs,* 16(6). Pp. 115–120.

Jonsen, A. R. (1997). *The Birth of Bioethics.* New York, London: Oxford University Press.

Jonsen, A. R., & Toulmin, S. (1998). *The Abuse of Casuistry.* Berkeley: University of California Press.

Joseph, J., & Deshpande, S. (1997). The Impact of Ethical Climate on Job Satisfaction of Nurses. *Health Care Manage Review,* 22(1). Pp. 76–81.

Journal of the American Medical Association. (1997). Medical News and Perspectives. *Journal of the American Medical Association,* 277. Pp. 1265–1268.

Juran, J. M., & Gryna, F. (1980). *Quality Planning and Analysis.* (2nd. ed.). New York: McGraw-Hill.

Kant, I. (1786; 1956). *Groundwork for the Metaphysic of Morals.* H. J. Paton (Trans.). New York: Harper Torchbooks.

Katz, J. P., & Paine, L. S. (1994). Levi Strauss & Co.: Global Sourcing. *Harvard University Graduate School of Business Administration Case # 9–395–f.* Boston: Harvard Business School Press, pp. 127–128.

Keeley, M. (1988). *A Social-Contract Theory of Organizations.* Notre Dame, IN: Notre Dame University Press.

Kleinke, J. P. (1998). Deconstructing the Columbia/HCA Investigation. *Health Affairs,* 17(2). Pp. 17–29.

Kotter, J. P., & Heskett, J. L. (1992). *Corporate Culture and Performance.* New York: Free Press.

Krajewski, L., & Ritzman, L. (1993). *Operations Management: Strategy and Analysis.* (3rd. ed.). Reading, MA: Addison-Wesley.

Kuczewski, M. G. (1997). *Fragmentation and Consensus: Communitarian and Casuist Bioethics.* Washington, DC: Georgetown University Press.

Kuhse, H. (1997). *Caring: Nurses, Women and Ethics.* Oxford: Blackwell's Publishing.

Ladd, J. (1970). Morality and the Ideal of Rationality in Formal Organizations. *Monist,* 54. Pp. 488–516.

Leake, C. (1927). *Percival's Medical Ethics.* Baltimore: Williams and Wilkins.

Lipson, E. H. (1993). What Are Purchasers Looking for in Managed Care Quality? *Topics in Health Care Finance,* 20(2). Pp. 1–9.

Luben, D. (1988). *Lawyers and Justice.* Princeton, NJ: Princeton University Press.

Lundberg, G.D. (1997). Editorial. *Journal of the American Medical Association,* 278. P. 1704.

May, L. (1987). *The Morality of Groups.* Notre Dame, IN: Notre Dame University Press.

Miller, F., & Fins, J. (1997). Clinical Pragmatism: A Method of Moral Problem Solving. *Kennedy Institute of Ethics Journal,* 7(2). Pp. 129–145.

Miller, R. B. (1996). *Casuistry and Modern Ethics: A Poetics of Practical Reasoning.* Chicago: University of Chicago Press.

Montoya, I. D., & Richard, A. J. (1994). A Comparative Study of Codes of Ethics in Health Care Facilities and Energy Companies. *Journal of Business Ethics*, 13. Pp. 713–717.

Moorthy, R. S., De George, R. T., Donaldson, T., Ellos, W. J., Solomon, R. C., & Textor, R. B. (1998). *Uncompromising Integrity: Motorola's Global Challenge*. Schaumburg, IL: Motorola University Press.

Mulligan, D., Shapiro, M., & Walrod, D. (1996). Managing Risk in Healthcare. *McKinsey Quarterly*, 3. Pp. 95–105.

National Coalition on Health Care. Available: http://www.nchc.org.

National Committee for Quality Assurance. (1997). *1997 Standards for Accreditation of Managed Care Organizations*. Washington, DC: NCQA, p. 85.

Navran, F. (1997). Twenty Steps to Total Ethics Management. Available: http://www.navran.com/Products/DTG/part07.html.

Neilson, N. (1998). An Overview of the Risk Management Process. *Risk Management*. Corvallis: Oregon State University College of Business. Ch. 1. Available: http://www.bus.orst.edu/faculty/neilson/rm/chapter1.htm.

Noddings, N. (1984). *Caring: A Feminine Ethics*. Berkeley: University of California Press.

Orr, R. D. (1992). Personal and Professional Integrity in Clinical Medicine. *Update*, 8(4). Pp. 1–3.

Ozar, D., & D. Sokol. (1994). *Dental Ethics by the Chairside*. St. Louis: Mosby-Year Book Co.

Peters, J. T., & Waterman, R. H., Jr. (1982). *In Search of Excellence*. Thorndike, ME: G. K. Hall & Co.

Phillips, M. (1992). Corporate Moral Personhood and Three Conceptions of the Corporation. *Business Ethics Quarterly*, 2. Pp. 435–459.

Phillips, R. (1997). Stakeholder Theory and a Principle of Fairness. *Business Ethics Quarterly*, 7. Pp. 51–66.

————. (Forthcoming). Normative Stakeholder Theory: Toward a Conception of Stakeholder Legitimacy.

Renz, D., & Eddy, W. (1996). Organization Ethics and Health Care: Building an Ethics Infrastructure for a New Era. *Bioethics Forum*, Summer 1996, 12(2). Pp. 29–39.

Rosenberg, C. (1987). *The Care of Strangers*. New York: Basic Books.

Rosner, D. (1982). *A Once Charitable Enterprise*. New York: Cambridge University Press.

Rothman, D. J. (1991). *Strangers at the Bedside*. New York: Basic Books, HarperCollins Publishers.

Schneider, B. (1975). Organizational Climates: An Essay. *Personnel Psychology*, 28. Pp. 447–479.

Schyve, Paul. (1995). Presentation to the Virginia Bioethics Network, Charlottesville, VA, October.

Scott, W. R. (1998). *Organizations: Rational, Natural, and Open Systems*. (4th. ed.). Upper Saddle River, NJ: Prentice-Hall.

Sen, A. (1987). *On Ethics and Economics*. Oxford: Basil Blackwell.

Siegler, M. (1982). Decision Making Strategy for Clinical-Ethical Problems in Medicine. *Archives of Internal Medicine*, 142. Pp. 2178–2179.

Siegler, M., Pellegrino, E. D., & Singer, P. A. (1990). Clinical Medical Ethics. *The Journal of Clinical Ethics*, 1(1). Pp. 5–9.

Simon, H. (1965). *Administrative Behavior*. (2nd. ed.). New York: Free Press.

Simmons, K. L. (1992). Managed Health Care: Right Idea—Wrong Rules. Ph.D. thesis, University of Texas at Austin.

Skocpol, T. (1995). The Rise and Resounding Demise of the Clinton Plan. *Health Affairs*, 14(1). Pp. 66–85.

Smith, A. (1759; 1976). *The Theory of Moral Sentiments*. A. L. Macfie and D. D. Raphael (Eds.). Oxford: Oxford University Press.

Smith, W. K., & Tedlow, R. S. (1989). James Burke: A Career in American Business. *Harvard University Graduate School of Business Administration Case #9-389-177*. Boston: Harvard Business School Press.

Solomon, R. (1992). *Ethics and Excellence*. New York: Oxford University Press.

Spencer, E. (1995). Economics, Managed Care, and Patient Advocacy. In J. Fletcher, P. Lombardo, M. F. Marshall, & F. Miller (Eds.), *Introduction to Clinical Ethics*. Frederick, MD: University Publishing Group, pp. 239–256.

———. (1997a). A New Role for Institutional Ethics Committees: Organizational Ethics. *Journal of Clinical Ethics*, 8(4). Pp. 372–376.

———. (1997b). Professional Ethics. In J. Fletcher, F. Miller, & M. F. Marshall (Eds.), *Introduction to Clinical Ethics*. (2nd. ed.). Frederick, MD: University Publishing Group. Pp. 287–300.

———. (1997c). *Recommendations for Guidelines on Procedures and Process to Address 'Organization Ethics' in Health Care Organizations (HCOs)*. Charlottesville, VA: Virginia Bioethics Network.

Starr, P. (1982). *The Social Transformation of American Medicine*. New York: Basic Books.

Thier, S., & Gelijns, A. (1998). Improving Health: The Reason Performance Measurement Matters. *Health Affairs*, 17(4). Pp. 26–28

Thomasma, D. (1978). Training in Medical Ethics: An Ethical Workup. *Forum on Medicine*, 1(9). Pp. 33–36.

Treviño, L. K., Weaver, G. R., Gibson, D. G., & Toffler, B. L. (1999). Managing Ethics and Legal Compliance: What Works and What Hurts? *California Management Review*, 41(2). Pp. 131–151.

U.S. Department of Justice. (1995). Sentencing of Organizations. *Federal Sentencing Guidelines*. Available: http://www.ussc.gov/guide/ch8web.htm.

———. (1999). *Health Care Fraud Report, Fiscal Years 1995–1996*. Available: http://www.usdoj.gov/opa/health/hcf1.htm.

Veatch, R. M. (1981). *A Theory of Medical Ethics*. New York: Basic Books.

Velasquez, M. (1983). Why Corporations Are Not Morally Responsible for Anything They Do. *Business and Professional Ethics Journal*, 2. Pp. 1–18.

———. (1998). *Business Ethics: Concepts and Cases*. (4th. ed.). Upper Saddle River, NJ: Prentice-Hall.

Victor, B., & Cullen, J. (1988). The Organizational Bases of Ethical Work Climates. *Administrative Science Quarterly*, 33. Pp. 101–125.

Virginia Health Maintenance Organizations Directory. (1997). P. 6.

Vogel, M. (1980). *The Invention of the Modern Hospital*. Chicago: University of Chicago Press.

Walzer, M. (1994). *Thick and Thin*. Notre Dame, IN: Notre Dame University Press.

Weaver, G. R, & Treviño, L. K. (1999). Attitudinal and Behavioral Outcomes of Corporate Ethics Programs: An Empirical Study of the Impact of Compliance and Values-Oriented Approaches. *Business Ethics Quarterly*, 9(2). Pp. 315–335.

Weick, K. (1974). Middle Range Theories of Social Systems. *Behavioral Science*, 19a. Pp. 357–367.

———. (1995). *Sensemaking in Organizations*. Thousand Oaks, CA: Sage.

Werhane, P. (1985). *Persons, Rights, and Corporations*. Englewood Cliffs, NJ: Prentice-Hall.

————. (1998a). Moral Imagination and Management Decision-Making. *Business Ethics Quarterly*, 8 (Special Issue). Pp. 75–98.

————. (1998b). Self-Interests, Roles and Some Limits to Role Morality. *Public Affairs Quarterly*, 12. Pp. 221–241.

Werhane, P., & J., Doering. (1995). Conflicts of Interest and Conflicts of Commitment. *Professional Ethics*, 4. Pp. 47–82.

Wicks, A., Gilbert, D., & Freeman, R. E. (1994). A Feminist Reinterpretation of the Stakeholder Concept. *Business Ethics Quarterly*, 4. Pp. 475–498.

Wilhelm, W. (1992). Changing Corporate Culture or Corporate Behavior? How to Change Your Company. *Academy of Management Executives*, 6(4). Pp. 72–77.

Williams, K., & Donnelly, P. (1982). *Medical Care Quality and the Public Trust*. Chicago: Pluribus Press.

Index

237